Gynecologic Disorders
of Children
and Adolescents

Clinical Practice of Gynecology

Michael S. Baggish, MD, *Series Editor*

Recent Issues

AIDS in Gynecology
Newton G. Osborne, Editor

Human Papillomavirus Infections
Barbara Winkler and Ralph Richart, Editors

Forthcoming Issues

DES Update
Kenneth L. Noller, Editor

Premalignant Lesions of the Lower Genital Tract
Albert Singer, Editor

Laser Endoscopy
Michael S. Baggish, Editor

Clinical Practice of
Gynecology

Series Editor: Michael S. Baggish, MD

Gynecologic Disorders of Children and Adolescents

Editor:

Donald Peter Goldstein, MD

Volume 1, Number 3, 1989

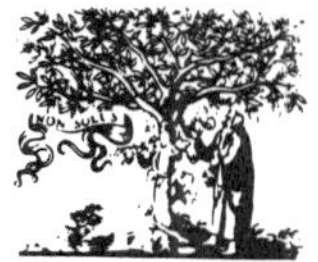

Elsevier

New York • Amsterdam • London

Clinical Practice of Gynecology is abstracted in *Excerpta Medica.*

Clinical Practice of Gynecology is published three times a year by Elsevier Science Publishing Co., Inc., 655 Avenue of the Americas, New York, NY 10010. Subscription price: institution $65.00, individual $55.00. Please add $19.00 for surface delivery outside the U.S., Canada, and Mexico. Claims for missing issues can be honored only up to three months for domestic addresses or six months for foreign addresses. Duplicate copies will not be mailed to replace ones lost through failure to notify Elsevier of change of address. Single copy and back volume information available on request.

Postmaster: please send address changes to *Clinical Practice of Gynecology*, Elsevier Science Publishing Co., Inc., 655 Avenue of the Americas, New York, NY 10010.

Please direct orders for this series, change of address, and claims for missing issues to: Journals Fulfillment Department, Elsevier Science Publishing Co., 655 Avenue of the Americas, New York, NY 10010.

Gynecologic Disorders of Children and Adolescents

CONTENTS

Gynecologic Disorders of Children and Adolescents

CONTRIBUTORS

MARIAN C. CRAIGHILL, MD, MPh, Staff Gynecologist, The Children's Hospital, Boston; Harvard Medical School, Boston, Massachusetts 02115

ANN JEANETTE DAVIS, MD, Fellow in Pediatric and Adolescent Gynecology, The Children's Hospital; Assistant Professor of Obstetrics and Gynecology, Tufts New England Medical Center, Boston, Massachusetts 02111

S. JEAN EMANS, MD, Associate Professor of Pediatrics, Harvard Medical School, Boston; Associate Chief, Division of Adolescent/Young Adult Medicine, The Children's Hospital, Boston, Massachusetts 02115

DONALD PETER GOLDSTEIN, MD, Assistant Clinical Professor of Obstetrics and Gynecology, Harvard Medical School, Boston; Chief, Division of Gynecology, The Children's Hospital, Boston, Massachusetts 02115

LAURENCE E. LUNDY, MD, Department of Obstetrics and Gynecology, Baystate Medical Center, Springfield, Massachusetts 01199

MAUREEN M. LYNCH, MD, Clinical Instructor in Pediatrics, Harvard Medical School; Department of Pediatrics, Harvard University Health Service; Staff Physician in the Gynecology Clinic, The Children's Hospital, Boston, Massachusetts 02115

JACQUES ROBERT MAILLOUX, MD, FRCP, McLaughlin Fellow in Pediatric and Adolescent Gynecology, The Children's Hospital, Boston, and Laval University, Quebec, Canada

M. JOAN MANSFIELD, MD, Instructor in Medicine, Harvard Medical School; Assistant in Medicine, The Children's Hospital, Boston, Massachusetts 02115

MARIETTA MURPHY, MD, Medical Director, Emergency Services, The Children's Hospital, Boston; Instructor in Pediatrics, Harvard Medical School, Boston, Massachusetts 02115

PAUL VON OEYEN, MD, Assistant Director, Maternal Fetal Medicine, William Beaumont Hospital, Royal Oak, Michigan 48072

VERONICA A. RAVNIKAR, MD, Assistant Professor in Obstetrics, Gynecology, and Reproductive Biology, Harvard Medical School; Staff Physician, Department of Obstetrics and Gynecology, Brigham and Women's Hospital, Boston, Massachusetts 02115

MITCHELL S. REIN, MD, Instructor in Obstetrics, Gynecology, and Reproductive Biology, Harvard Medical School, Boston, Massachusetts 02115

JANE SHARE, MD, Fellow in Radiology, Harvard Medical School; Department of Radiology, The Children's Hospital, Boston, Massachusetts 02115

RITA TEELE, MD, Assistant Professor of Radiology, Harvard Medical School; Staff Radiologist, The Children's Hospital; Consultant in Neonatal Radiology, Brigham and Women's Hospital, Boston, Massachusetts 02115

CHAPTER 1

Examination of the Pediatric and Adolescent Female

S. Jean Emans, MD

Medical care of the child and adolescent often involves the evaluation of gynecologic complaints. Knowledge of the approach to the child and correct techniques for examination is essential to the practicing physician.

GYNECOLOGIC EXAMINATION OF THE PREPUBERTAL CHILD

The gynecologic examination of the prepubertal girl is quite different from the traditional speculum examination of the adolescent and adult woman. Before the child is asked to undress, the confidence of the child should be gained by the examiner speaking with both the parent and child. Involving the child in choices such as the color of the gown or type of flashlight can be very helpful. A running conversation about toys, television shows, or siblings can aid in putting the child at ease. The parent should be visible to the child or even holding her hand if needed. The physician may need to slow the tempo of the examination for the child who has been molested or has had previous painful gynecologic assessment.

Because gynecologic problems may be associated with systemic illnesses or skin diseases in the child, a complete physical examination should be done for signs of puberty, adenopathy, pharyngitis, hernias, and skin disease. The genital examination should include inspection of the external genitalia with the child supine (feet together, knees apart) and by the labia pulled gently forward (Figure 1-1).[1,2] The normal clitoral glans is 3 mm in width. Friability of the posterior forchette as the labia are separated can occur in children with vulvitis and/or history of sexual abuse.[3] Although it is rare in the prepubertal child, lichen sclerosis produces a characteristic

Clinical Practice of Gynecology: **3,** 1–15, 1989
© 1989 Elsevier Science Publishing Co., Inc.
655 Avenue of the Americas, New York, NY 10010
ISSN 1043-3198/89/$3.50

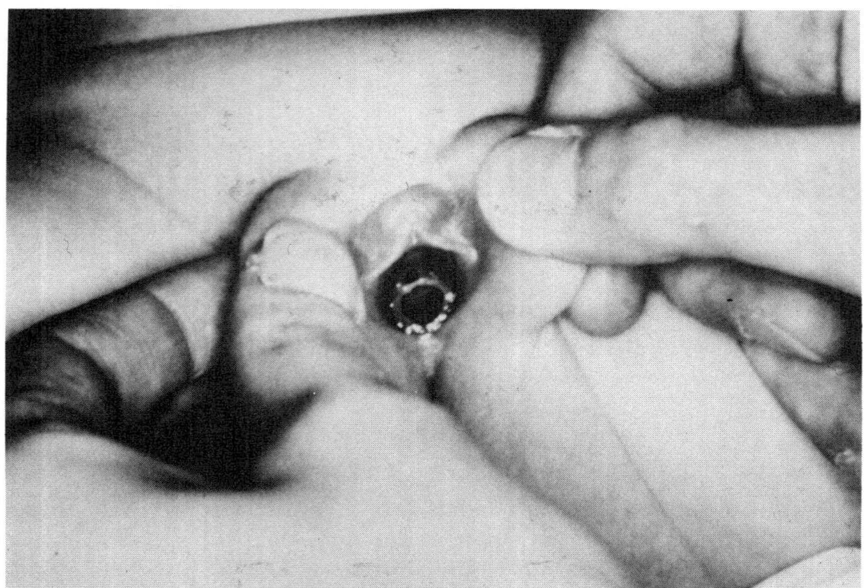

FIGURE 1-1 Examination of the vulva and hymen of a child, pulling the labia gently forward (from ref. 2, with permission of Pediatr Rev).

atrophic, white figure-of-eight pattern around the vagina and anus, often accompanied by excoriations, macerations, secondary infection, and small hemorrhages (Figure 1-2). With the child in the supine position, the anterior vagina can be visualized, and the hymenal ring can be examined by using the magnification and light of an otoscope for evidence of lacerations, attenuation, or synechiae suggestive of sexual abuse. Normal hymens are shown in Figures 1-3 through 1-5.

After initial inspection of vulva and introitus, the physician should examine the child in the knee-chest position to allow visualization of the upper vagina and cervix using an otoscope (Figure 1-6).[1,2,4] Other methods that have been used for visualization of the vagina include placing the child in lithotomy position or on the mother's lap and inserting a small veterinary otoscope speculum or a hysteroscope. Some physicians have found that for a 2- or 3-year-old child, having the mother on the table in stirrups with the child resting on her lower abdomen with legs apart can result in a more relaxed examination.

If the presenting complaint is vulvovaginitis, a specific diagnosis is more likely in girls with visible discharge during the examination.[5] If the initial examination is normal, the child has no visible discharge, and the history is not suggestive of a specific infection, the child can be treated with sitz baths and appropriate hygiene. In the child with a persistent or purulent discharge, cultures and "wet preps" should be obtained with the use of a

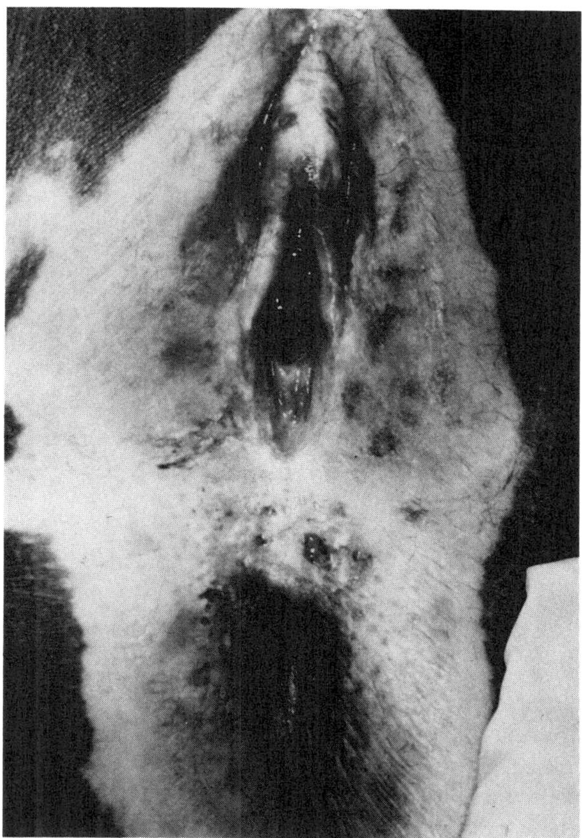

FIGURE 1-2 Lichen sclerosis in a prepubertal child (from ref. 1, 3rd ed, with permission of Little, Brown and Company).

small plastic Clinitest dropper or a saline-moistened Calgiswab. If multiple samples are needed, a small amount of saline can be squeezed into the vagina with the Clinitest dropper or a small feeding tube or urethral catheter attached to a syringe and aspirated back. Appropriate cultures should be done for *N. gonorrhoeae, C. trachomatis,* and other pathogens. Hammerschlag's data, the normal flora of the vagina, are shown in Table 1-1.[6] More data is clearly needed because of the wide range of ages, including pubertal and prepubertal, and the small number of subjects examined in an inner-city hospital. In children with vaginal itching or white discharge, a swab can be streaked directly onto Biggy agar to look for *Candida.* "Wet preps," which usually show white cells in the child with vaginitis, are much less helpful in making a specific diagnosis than is the case in the adolescent or adult woman with vaginitis. A Gram stain of a purulent discharge can be

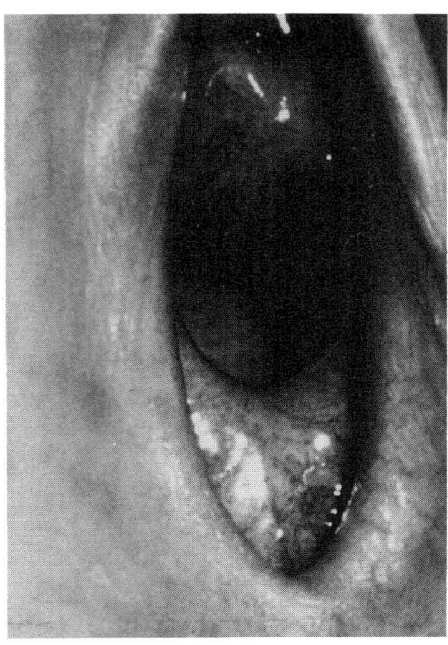

FIGURE 1-3 Crescent hymen (from ref. 2, with permission of Pediatr Rev).

helpful in making a specific diagnosis than is the case in the adolescent or adult woman with vaginitis. A Gram stain of a purulent discharge can be helpful in making a presumptive diagnosis of *N. gonorrhoeae,* although culture is always necessary because occasionally other *Neisseria* may cause vaginitis in the prepubertal child. If possible, girls with suspected sexual abuse or persistent symptoms should have a vaginal culture obtained for *C. trachomatis.* A dacron (male) urethral swab can be used to obtain epithelial cells from the vagina.

Girls with vulvar and anal pruritis should be screened for pinworms. Because the rectal exam is sometimes uncomfortable for the child, it should be performed last. The child should be in lithotomy position with knees apart and feet together. A bimanual rectal–abdominal examination can be used to detect a mass or foreign body and to milk any discharge forward. X-ray studies and ultrasonography of the abdomen and pelvis are rarely indicated except when the question of a tumor, an ovarian cyst, an abscess, or an ectopic urethra is raised. For children with whom an adequate examination is not possible because of poor cooperation, or the vagina does not gape open in knee–chest position, brief assessment under general anesthesia may be necessary. This is particularly true in girls with vaginal bleeding, persistent discharge, and those under the age of 2 years.

The prepubertal girl is particularly susceptible to nonspecific irritation of the vulvovaginal area but can also have specific infection from respiratory

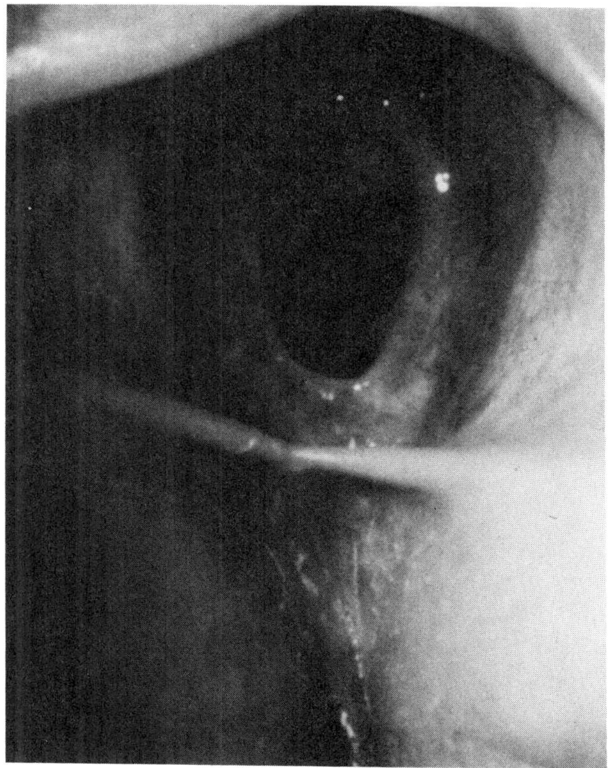

FIGURE 1-4 Annular hymen (from ref. 1, 3rd ed, with permission of Little, Brown and Company).

or enteric pathogens or sexually acquired organisms. "Nonspecific" vulvovaginitis is the diagnosis of 25–75% of children seen in referral centers for evaluation of vulvovaginitis.[4,7–9] This term applies to children whose vaginal cultures grow normal flora or gram-negative enteric organisms, usually *E. coli,* and who have no other etiology for the vaginitis. Nonspecific vulvovaginal irritation can result from irritants and allergic contacts, pinworm infestation, the wearing of tight-fitting nylon clothes, obesity, masturbation, reflux of urine into the vagina, and sexual abuse. It appears that either a high hymenal opening, which does not allow normal vaginal drainage, or a gaping hymenal ring, which allows easy contamination of the vagina, can predispose to nonspecific vaginitis. It is possible that children who are susceptible to recurrent vulvovaginitis may have other, as yet undefined factors that promote adherence of bacteria to vulvar epithelial cells. The role of toxigenic or invasive strains of *E. coli* and other enteric organisms, such as Campylobacter, has not been investigated.

A list of specific infection seen in prepubertal children is included in

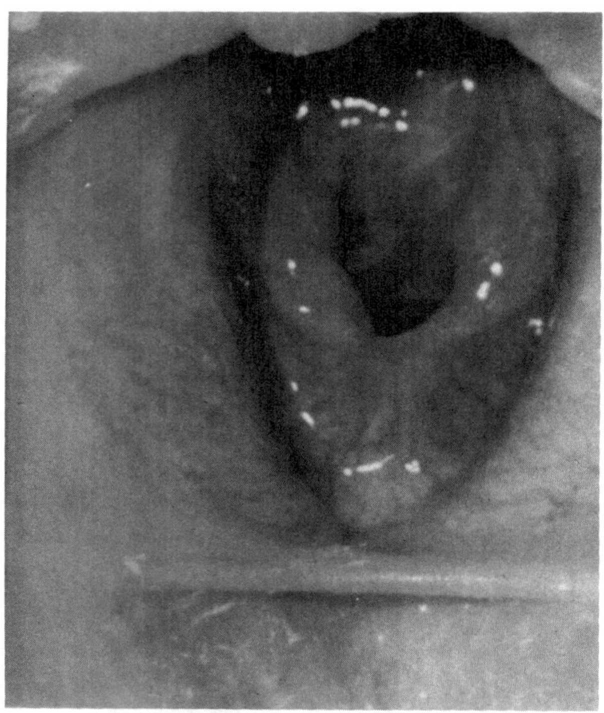

FIGURE 1-5 Redundant hyman (from ref. 1, 3rd ed, with permission of Little, Brown and Company).

Table 1-2. *Staphylococcus aureus* and *Hemophilus influenzae* can occur as normal flora but appear to be responsible for some cases of vaginitis as well. The latter may occur with impetiginous lesions in the vulva and buttocks.

The isolation of *Gardnerella vaginalis* from the vagina of prepubertal girls appears to be more likely in sexually abused girls than control patients or patients with genitourinary complaints.[10] However, Bartley[10] did not find any association of this organism with vaginal erythema or discharge.

The presence of *C. trachomatis* in a vagina of prepubertal children has been recently associated with a history of sexual abuse.[11,12] Although some infants can be expected to acquire vaginal colonization with *C. trachomatis* at birth from a mother with endocervical infection, persistence for more than 12–24 months is unlikely.[13] Other causes of vulvovaginal complaints are vaginal foreign bodies, vaginal and cervical polyps and tumors, urethral prolapse, systemic illnesses (measles, chickenpox, mononucleosis, Crohn's, scarlet fever), anomalies (eg, ectopic ureter or obstructed double vagina with a fistula) and vulvar skin disease. Occasionally, children have psycho-

Table 1-1. Normal Flora of the Vagina in Girls 2 Months to 15 Years*

Organism	% of Patients
Diphtheroids	78
Staphylococcus epidermis	73
Hemolytic streptococci	39
Lactobacilli	39
Nonhemolytic streptococci	34
Escherichia coli	34
Klebsiella	15
Group D Streptococcus	8.5
Staphylococcus aureus	7
Haemophilus influenzae	5
Pseudomonas aeruginosa	5
Proteus	5
Gardnerella vaginalis	13.5

*From reference 6.

somatic vaginal complaints of itching, or "tickling," which usually precipitate great concern from the parent.

For children with symptoms of vulvitis, a brief history and external examination in the office and instructions to the parent on improved hygiene, avoidance of irritants, and/or the treatment of pinworms is all that is needed. Any child with persistent purulent or recurrent vaginal discharge deserves a thorough gynecologic assessment. Itching and redness are usually nonspecific signs of irritation. Behavioral changes and somatic symptoms, such as abdominal pain, headaches, and enuresis, may suggest sexual abuse. Information on the caretaker should be elicited. The child should be asked both at the time of history and later during the exam about a possibility of abuse.

Table 1-2. Etiology of Vulvovaginitis in the Prepubertal Child*

Nonspecific Vulvovaginitis
Specific infections: group A *β-Streptococcus, Streptococcus pneumoniae, Neisseria meningitidis, Candida, Shigella, Staphylococcus aureus, Haemophilus influenzae, Neisseria gonorrhoeae, Condyloma accuminatum, Herpes Simplex, Trichomonas, Chlamydia trachomatis, Gardnerella vaginalis*
Pinworms
Foreign body
Polyps, tumors
Systemic illness: measles, chickenpox, scarlet fever, Stephen-Johnson syndrome
Vulvar skin disease: seborrhea, psoriasis, atopic dermatitis, lichen sclerosis, scabies
Trauma
Psychosomatic vaginal complaints
Miscellaneous: draining pelvic abscess, prolapsed urethra, ectopic ureter

*From Emans SJ: Vulvovaginitis in the child and adolescent. Pediatr Rev 1986;8:13.

Table 1-3. Treatment of Vulvovaginitis in the Prepubertal Child

Etiology	Treatment
Group A β-Streptococcus S. pneumoniae	Pen VK 125–250 mg. q.i.d. × 10 days
C. trachomatis	Erythromycin 50 mg/kg/d p.o. × 10 days
N. gonorrhoeae	Ceftriaxone 125 mg (<45 kg) Ceftriaxone 250 mg (>45 kg)
Candida	Topical mycostatin, miconazole, or clotrimazole cream
Shigella	Trimethoprim/sulfamethoxazole 8 mg/40mg/kg/day p.o. × 7 days
Staphylococcus aureus	Cephalexin 25–50 mg/kg/day × 7–10 days Dicloxacillin 12.5–25 mg/kg/day × 7–10 days
H. influenzae	Amoxicillin 20–40 mg/kg/day × 7 days
Trichomonas	Metronidazole 125 mg (15 mg/kg/day) t.i.d. × 7–10 days

Treatment of nonspecific vulvovaginitis includes hygiene; avoidance of nylon tights, leotards, blue jeans, sleepers, and wool; double rinsing of cotton underwear; tepid sitz baths; and hand washing. After the bath, the child or mother should pat the vulva dry. A 2–3-day course of topical hydrocortisone can alleviate the discomfort of girls who have recurrent vulvar erythema and pain (without vaginitis), usually related to local irritation. In persistent cases of nonspecific vaginitis, a 10-day course of oral antibiotics, such as amoxicillin or a cephalosporin, may clear the discharge. Rarely, topical estrogen is warranted to thicken the vagina and vulva to make it more resistant to infection.

The treatment of specific infections is outlined in Table 1-3. *Candida* vaginal infections are treated with topical nystatin, miconazole nitrate, or clotrimazole cream because intravaginal medications are rarely necessary or practical. Since *Candida* vaginal infections are uncommon in prepubertal girls except after a course of broad spectrum antibiotics, screening for diabetes in this age group is important. Since the parent frequently has concerns about the cause of the vaginitis that are out of proportion to the problem, it is important to do a careful examination and outline a treatment program for the child and parent.

LABIAL ADHESIONS IN THE PREPUBERTAL GIRL

Agglutination of the labia minora, termed labial adhesions, occurs primarily in young girls between age 3 months and 6 years (Figure 1-7). Adhesions may occasionally occur later or persist to the time of puberty. It is possible, although unproven, that hygiene and vulvar irritation can cause a small adhesion to result in near total fusion. It has been suggested but not proven that fondling and the irritation from sexual abuse may predispose the older girl to labial agglutination.[14]

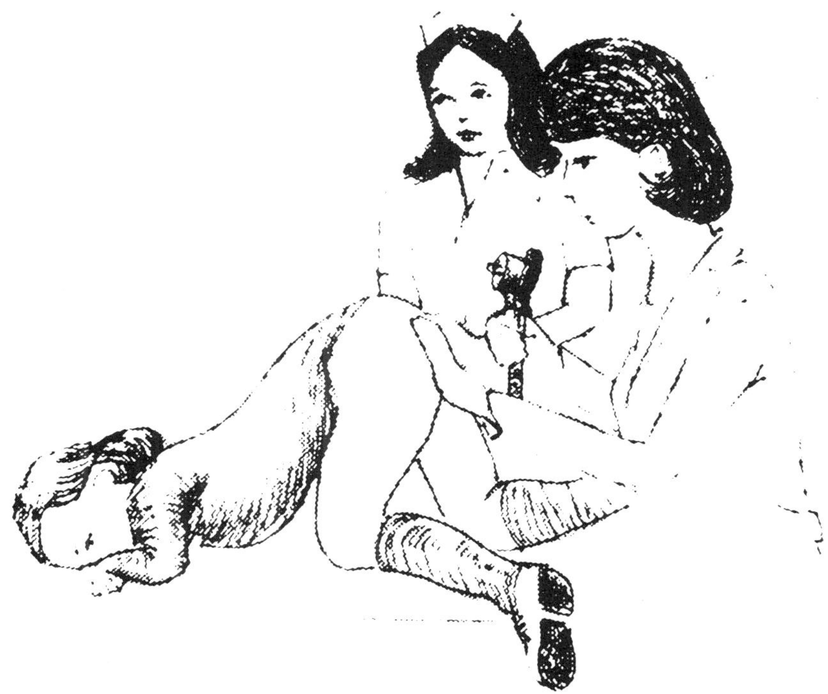

FIGURE 1-6 Knee-chest position for visualization of the vagina and cervix in the prepubertal child (from ref. 1, with permission of Little, Brown and Company).

The diagnosis of labial adhesions is made by visual inspection of the vulva. The treatment of labial adhesions remains controversial. Spontaneous separation may occur, particularly with small labial adhesions at the posterior forchette and with estrogenization at puberty. If the opening in the agglutination is large enough for good vaginal and urinary drainage, lubrication of the labia with a bland ointment such as A&D ointment and gentle separation by the mother over several weeks may be helpful. For adhesions that impair vaginal or urinary drainage, the most effective treatment is application of an estrogen-containing cream (Premarin) twice daily for 2–4 weeks. After separation has occurred, the labia should be maintained apart by daily baths, good hygiene, and the application of a bland ointment (such as A&D ointment) at bedtime for 6–12 months. Forced separation is traumatic to the child, and adhesions frequently recur.

GYNECOLOGIC EVALUATION OF THE ADOLESCENT

The gynecologic evaluation of the adolescent needs to be undertaken with special sensitivity. After an explanation of the pelvic exam, the adolescent

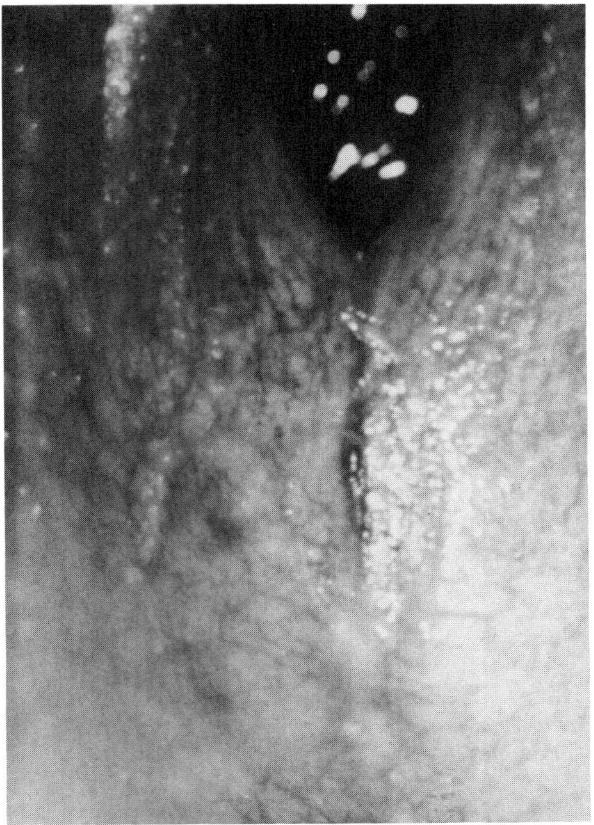

FIGURE 1-7 Labial adhesion (from ref. 1, with permission of Little, Brown and Company).

should be given a gown and drape. A general physical examination, including a breast examination, is done first. The pelvic exam begins with inspection of the external genitalia; the Tanner stage of pubic hair and the size of the clitoris should be noted. The width of the normal glans is less than 5 mm. The size of the hymenal opening and degree of estrogenization should be evaluated. Each part of the examination should be discussed again during the actual procedure. Examining adolescents can be much more time-consuming than examining adult women, but a positive first experience with pelvic examination can set the tone for future assessments. The patient needs to feel in control of the tempo and type of evaluation and needs to understand why each part is important in the diagnosis of her problem. The examination should be modified to fit the patient. For example, in a virginal young teenager with a tight hymen and white vaginal discharge, a small

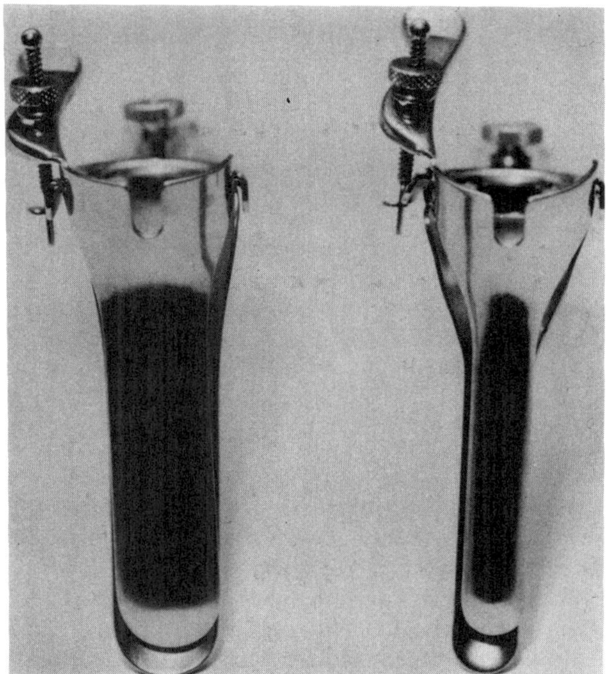

FIGURE 1-8 Pederson (left) and Hoffman (right) specula.

amount of the discharge can be obtained for "wet preps" and culture on Biggy agar by the gentle insertion of a saline-moistened, cotton-tipped applicator through the hymenal ring. The virginal adolescent with pelvic pain or dysmenorrhea may require only an inspection of the hymenal opening and a careful rectoabdominal bimanual palpation. Too often, no examination is done, and pathology is missed because the adolescent is considered too young. Because assumptions about sexual activity are often made on the basis of race or social class, the diagnosis of sexually transmitted infections can be delayed markedly in teenagers. Ultrasonography is useful but should not be considered a substitute for careful history and physical examination.

Speculum examinations are possible in most girls. If the hymen is 1 cm wide, a virginal speculum, the Huffman speculum, can be gently inserted. In sexually active adolescents and virginal adolescents with a larger hymenal opening, the Pederson speculum offers optimal visualization of the cervix (Figure 1-8). Because of the high incidence of sexually transmitted infections in adolescents, at least annual Papanicolaou smears and cultures for *N. gonorrhoeae* and *C. trachomatis* should be obtained. The prevalence of *C. trachomatis* cervical infections in adolescents range from 5–23% in nonpregnant teenagers and 21–27% in pregnant adolescents.[15–21]

In the adolescent, the appearance of any vaginal discharge should be noted, and the sample of the discharge should be tested with pH paper. "Wet preps" and whiff test should be performed in patients with symptoms, abnormal discharge, or a pH greater than 4.5.

After the speculum is removed, the uterus and adnexae should be palpated by bimanual one- or two-finger vaginal–abdominal examination. A recto–vaginal–abdominal examination allows palpation of a retroverted uterus and uterosacral ligaments.

VULVOVAGINITIS IN THE ADOLESCENT

Similar to the adult woman, the adolescent with vaginitis is likely to have a specific etiology for her discharge: *Candida,* trichomonas, or bacterial vaginosis. The young virginal adolescent of 12 or 13 years old who complains of discharge most likely has leukorrhea (normal desquamation of cells and mucus) or *Candida* vaginitis. In contrast, the sexually active adolescent may have one or more sexually transmitted infections (see Chapter 8). *Chlamydia trachomatis* and *N. gonorrhoeae* can cause cervicitis, which may present as vaginal discharge. Patients with primary herpes simplex may have cervical as well as vulvar lesions that can cause discharge. In addition, adolescents with primary herpes may have coexisting *Candida* vaginitis. The possibility of a foreign body, especially a retained tampon, should be considered in adolescents with a foul-smelling, bloody vaginal discharge. Occasionally, a partially obstructed Mullerian anomaly will present with foul-smelling discharge starting with menarche.

The diagnosis of vaginitis is made from the history, the appearance of the discharge, the "wet preps," vaginal pH, and cultures. *Candida* vaginitis usually presents with a white discharge and itching, especially prominent before and after the menstrual period. Predisposing factors include diabetes, use of antibiotics, immunosuppressive drugs, corticosteroids, pregnancy, obesity, and tight-fitting clothes. The vulva may be erythematous and the discharge thick, white, and curdy. The KOH prep has a sensitivity of 80–90% in the symptomatic patient. A Biggy culture should be obtained in questionable cases, since otherwise adolescents with nonspecific or allergic itching may tend to be treated recurrently with antifungal creams.[22, 23]

Trichomonas infections typically cause an irritating odorous discharge; dysuria may be present. Flagellated organisms and polymorphonuclear leukocytes are seen on wet prep in greater than 75% of symptomatic women. However, in patients seen in sexually transmitted diseases (STD) clinics without regard to symptoms, the wet smear detects only about 50% of those detected by culture. The Papanicolaou smear appears to detect 33% to 79% of those found on culture, but false positives occcur. Cultures are

Table 1-4. Treatment of the Adolescent with Vaginitis

Candida	Clotrimazole 500 mg vaginal tab × 1 day, or
	Clotrimazole 200 mg vaginally HS × 3 days, or
	Clotrimazole 1% cream HS × 7 days, or
	Miconazole 2% cream HS × 7 days, or
	Miconazole 200 mg vaginally HS × 3, or
	Butoconazole cream HS × 3, or
	Mycostatin cream b.i.d. × 14 days
Trichomonas	Metronidazole 2 gm single dose
Bacterial vaginosis	Metronidazole 500 mg b.i.d. × 7 days, or
	Clindomycin 300 mg b.i.d. × 7 days

the most sensitive method of detection. [24–27] Monoclonal antibody staining of direct specimens looks promising.[28]

Bacterial vaginosis, also termed *Gardnerella vaginalis*-associated vaginosis or nonspecific vaginitis, has been the subject of much controversy over the years because of the occurrence of *G. vaginalis* and clue cells in asymptomatic women. Shafer[29] reported that approximately one-third of virginal adolescent girls and two-thirds of sexually experienced girls had *G. vaginalis* detected by vaginal cultures. Current theory based on the work of Holmes and associates suggests that bacterial vaginosis involves a complex alteration in microbial flora with an increase in *G. vaginalis* and in anaerobic bacteria, a decrease in lactobacilli, and an increase in organic acids.[23] Thus, the diagnosis in the symptomatic patient should be based on three of four criteria: 1) a gray-to-white homogeneous thin discharge adherent to vaginal walls, 2) vaginal pH>4.5, 3) a positive "whiff test," and 4) clue cells. The absence of lactobacillus on wet preps or Gram stain and the presence of gram-variable coccobacilli and curved gram-negative rods provides confirming evidence.[30,31]

Treatment for vaginitis is outlined in Table 1-4. Because of concern about toxicity, ketoconazole should probably not be used in the adolescent with recurrent *Candida* vaginitis until more data is available. Patients with recurrent infections should have a careful history to look for sources and factors of reinfection, including douche equipment, partners, medication, and screening for diabetes. Treatment of trichomonas should include the sexual partner. Although reinfection is usually the cause of "persistent" trichomonas, rare trichomonas isolates have acquired significant resistance to metronidazole.[32] The most effective dosage of metronidazole for bacterial vaginosis is still under study.[33,34] Clindamycin orally is an alternative for women with bacterial vaginosis. The diagnosis of a sexually transmitted infection should lead the physician to do sensitive counseling about abstinence, monogomy, barrier methods, and AIDS.

REFERENCES

1. Emans SJ, Goldstein DP: Pediatric and adolescent gynecology, 3rd ed. Boston: Little, Brown and Company, 1990.
2. Emans SJ: Vulvovaginitis in children and adolescents. Pediatrics in Review 1986;8:12.
3. Emans SJ, Wood ER, Flagg NT, et al: Genital findings in sexually abused, symptomatic and asymptomatic, girls. Pediatrics 1987;79:778.
4. Emans SJ, Goldstein DP: The gynecologic examination of the prepubertal child with vulvovaginitis: Use of the knee–chest position. Pediatrics 1980;65:758.
5. Paradise JE, Compos JM, Friedman HM, et al: Vulvovaginitis in premenarchal girls: Clinical features and diagnostic evaluation. Pediatrics 1982;70:193.
6. Hammerschlag MR, Albert S, Rosner I, et al: Microbiology of the vagina in children: Normal and potentially pathogenic organisms. Pediatrics 1978;68:57.
7. Altchek A: Pediatric vulvovaginitis. J Reprod Med 1984; 29:359.
8. Capraro VJ: Vulvovaginitis and other local lesions of the vulva. Clin Obstet Gynecol 1974;1:533.
9. Heller RH, Joseph JH, David HJ: Vulvovaginitis in the premenarchal child. J Pediatr 1969;74:370.
10. Bartley DL, Morgan L, Rimsza ME: *Gardnerella vaginalis* in prepubertal girls. Am J Dis Child 1987;141:1014.
11. Ingram DL, White ST, Occhiuti AC, et al: Childhood vaginal infections: Association of *Chlamydia trachomatis* with sexual contact. Pediatr Infect Dis 1986;5:226.
12. Fuster CD, Neinstein LS: Vaginal *Chlamydia trachomatis* prevalence in sexually abused prepubertal girls. Pediatrics 1987;79:235.
13. Schacter J, Grossman M, Sweet RL, et al: Prospective study of preinatal transmission of *Chlamydia trachomatis.* JAMA 1986;255:3374.
14. Berkowitz CD, Elvik SL, Logan MK: Labial fusion in prepubescent girls: A marker for sexual abuse? Am J Obstet Gynecol 1987;156:16.
15. Shafer, M-A, Beck A, Blain B, et al: *Chlamydia trachomatis:* Important relationships to race, contraception, lower genital tract infection, and Papanicolaou smear. J Pediatr 1984;104:141.
16. Chacko MR: *Chlamydia trachomatis* infection in sexually active adolescents: Prevalence and risk factors. Pediatrics 1984;73:836.
17. Skjeldestad FE, Dalen A: The prevalence of *C. trachomatis* in the cervix of pregnant women, and its consequence for the outcome of pregnancy. Scand J Prim Health Care 1986;4:209.
18. Fisher M, Swenson PO, Risucci D, et al: *Chlamydia trachomatis* in suburban adolescents. J Pediatr 1987;111:617.
19. McCormack WM, Alpert S, McComb DE, et al: Fifteen-month follow-up study of women infected with *Chlamydia trachomatis.* N Engl J Med 1979;300:123.
20. Khurana CM, Deddish PA, del Mundo F: Prevalence of *C. trachomatis* in the pregnant cervix. Obstet Gynecol 1985;66:241.
21. Fraser GJ, Rettig PJ, Kaplan DW: Prevalence of cervical *Chlamydia trachomatis* and *Neisseria gonorrhoeae* in female adolescents. Pediatrics 1983;71:333.
22. Eschenbach DA: Vaginal infections. Clin Obstet Gynecol 1983;26:1.
23. Holmes KK. Lower genital tract infections in women: Cystitis/urethritis, vulvovaginitis, and cervicitis. In Holmes KK, Mardh P, Sparling PF, et al, eds. *Sexually transmitted diseases*, 2nd ed. New York: McGraw-Hill, 1990.
24. Fouts AC, Kraus SJ: *Trichomonas vaginalis:* Reevaluation of its clinical presentation and laboratory diagnosis. J Infect Dis 1980;141:137.
25. Rein MF, Müller M: *Trichomonas vaginalis* and trichomoniosis. In Holmes KK, Mardh P, Sparling PF, et al, eds. *Sexually transmitted diseases*, 2nd ed. New York: McGraw-Hill, 1990.

26. Spence MR, Hollander DH, Smith J, et al: The clinical and laboratory diagnosis of *Trichomonas vaginalis* infection. Sex Transm Dis 1980;7:168.
27. Mason PR, Super H, Fripp PJ: Comparison of four techniques for the routine diagnosis of *Trichomonas vaginalis* infection. J Clin Pathol 1976;29:154.
28. Krieger JN, Tam MR, Stevens CE, et al: Diagnosis of trichomonas. JAMA 1988; 259:1223.
29. Shafer MA, Sweet RL, Ohm-Smith MS, et al: Microbiology of the lower genital tract in postmenarchal adolescent girls: Differences by sexual activity, contraception, and presence of nonspecific vaginitis. J Pediatr 1985;107:974.
30. Spiegel CA, Amsel R, Eschenbach D, et al: Anaerobic bacteria in nonspecific vaginitis. N Engl J Med 1980;303:601.
31. Amsel R, Totten PA, Spiegel CA, et al: Nonspecific vaginitis: Diagnostic criteria and microbial and epidemiologic associations. Am J Med 1983;74:14.
32. Muller M, Miengasser J, Miller W: Three metronidazole-resistant strains of *Trichomonas vaginalis* from the U.S. Am J Obstet Gynecol 1980;138:808.
33. Minkowski WL, Baker CJ, Alleyne D, et al: Single oral dose metronidazole therapy for *Gardnerella vaginalis* vaginitis in adolescent females. J Adolesc Health Care 1983;4:113–116.
34. Jerve F, Berdol TB, Bohman P, et al: Metronidazole in the treatment of nonspecific vaginitis (NSV). Br J Vener Dis 1984;60:171.

CHAPTER 2

Delayed Puberty

M. Joan Mansfield, MD

Puberty is the final phase of childhood growth and development during which a series of alterations in hormonal patterns result in the physical and psychologic maturation of the child into an adult who is capable of sexual and reproductive function.

An understanding of the normal variation in patterns of growth and pubertal development is the most important step in approaching disorders of puberty. The obvious physical changes of puberty are alterations in statural growth, body composition, and the appearance of secondary sexual characteristics. These physical changes are accompanied by an increased production of androgens by the adrenal glands, by estrogen and androgen production by the ovaries, and by a rise in growth hormone secretion from the pituitary. Statural growth that has been very rapid in utero decelerates during the first several years of postnatal life to reach an average rate of 5–6 cm per year during midchildhood. A child who grows less than 4 cm per year during this period should be evaluated to exclude an endocrinopathy or chronic disease. Statural growth rate is quite sensitive to small amounts of estrogen and begins to increase in many girls before any evidence of secondary sexual development is present. This pubertal growth spurt begins gradually at about age 9 and reaches a peak by age 12. Statural growth usually slows by the time menarche is reached at an average age of 12.8 years in the United States. Final height is determined by both the growth rate and the time available for growth. The gonadal sex steroids both increase the rate of growth and signal the beginning of the end of growth as epiphyses fuse under the influence of estrogen. Statural growth is virtually complete in females at a skeletal age of 15 years. Generally, a girl who develops somewhat early has a more exuberant growth spurt than her later-

Clinical Practice of Gynecology: **3,** 16–30, 1989

ISSN 1043-3198/89/$3.50   655 Avenue of the Americas, New York, NY 10010 developing counterpart, so that final height may be similar in individuals with very different tempos of pubertal development. An increase in weight accompanies the increase in height, and body composition continues to change throughout late childhood and adolescence. By age 18, women carry an average of 28% of their body weight as fat, about twice the fat stores of men. Men have a greater increase in muscle mass peaking in late adolescence, and they achieve a final muscle mass about one and one-half times that of women.

The first sign of secondary sexual development is breast budding in 85% of girls. Breast budding begins at an average age of 10.5–11 years and may be initially unilateral. Breast development is completed in about 4 years. Menarche usually occurs at Tanner B3–B4, about 2 years after the onset of breast development. Pubic hair usually lags 6 months behind breast development, appearing at an average age of 11–12; however, in about 15% of girls, pubic hair may be the first sign of puberty. This is most often a normal variant, although some of these individuals may have an excess of androgens that may cause hirsutism and persistent menstrual irregularity in later adolescence.

There is considerable individual variation in the timing of normal puberty. The first signs of secondary sexual development occur between the ages of 8 and 13 in 98.8% of girls. A girl who has no development by age 13 has delayed puberty by definition, since she is 2.5 standard deviations beyond the norm. This warrants an evaluation to exclude a pathologic cause of pubertal delay. Constitutional delay of puberty occurs less commonly in girls than in boys and is a diagnosis of exclusion. A girl who has not had menarche by age 16 or 4 years after the onset of breast development has delayed menarche that should be investigated.

The first hormonal change accompanying the pubertal process is adrenarche. In fetal life, the zona reticularis of the adrenal gland is well developed and secretes androgens that are converted to estrogens by the placenta. After birth, this zone regresses, and adrenal androgen levels fall. In midchildhood, the zona reticularis again enlarges and becomes continuous, and levels of adrenal androgens rise. Cortisol production rate for body size is not altered. During adrenarche, activity of the microsomal enzyme P450c17 increases, resulting in greater amounts of the androgens dehydroepiandrosterone and androstendione. Other adrenal enzyme systems may be involved as well. There is considerable individual variation in the timing of adrenarche, but levels of the adrenal androgen metabolite dehydroepiandrosterone sulfate usually increase by 6–8 years of age, well before secondary sexual development becomes apparent.

The hypothalamic–pituitary–gonadal axis is very active in boys in utero and in the first few months of postnatal life. The gonads are usually less active in utero in girls, but pulsatile LH patterns similar to those seen in puberty have been documented in young female infants as well as in males.

Infantile ovaries visualized by ultrasound or at autopsy often show many small cysts, as follicles develop in an anovulatory pattern reminiscent of polycystic ovaries. Premature thelarche, or isolated breast budding without growth acceleration in the first 2 years of life, is a frequent and usually self-limited accompaniment of this ovarian activity. By the age of 2–4, the hypothalamic–pituitary–ovarian axis is normally well suppressed by mechanisms as yet undescribed. This allows the relatively prolonged childhood of humans and other higher primates. Puberty represents a reawakening of the hypothalamic–pituitary–gonadal axis.

The trigger for the escape of gonadotropin-releasing hormone (GnRH) from inhibition that allows puberty to proceed remains unknown. Pulsatile release of GnRH from the hypothalamus is reflected in luteinizing hormone (LH) and, less clearly, follicle-stimulating hormone (FSH) synthesis and release from the pituitary, which in turn trigger activation of the gonads. Early in puberty, LH and FSH pulsations occur primarily during sleep. A girl who is in the early stages of normal puberty may have an estradiol level less than 20 pg/mL and daytime levels of LH and FSH in the prepubertal range. FSH levels and FSH response to exogenous GnRH often exceeds LH in the early stages of female puberty when estrogen levels are low.

CENTRAL CAUSES OF DELAYED PUBERTY

Interference with pulsatile GnRH release, pituitary response to GnRH, or ovarian response to pituitary gonadotropins results in absence or interruption of the progression of puberty. Central causes of delayed puberty result in inhibition of normal GnRH release from the hypothalamus. Central causes of pubertal disruption include chronic disease, poor nutrition, intensive exercise, certain endocrinopathies, and the use of drugs, such as opiates.

The most common central cause of pubertal delay is poor nutrition. This often occurs in the presence of a chronic childhood illness interfering with the absorption of food or increasing caloric demands in excess of food intake. Cystic fibrosis, inflammatory bowel disease, and celiac disease are examples. Usually the diagnosis is made on the basis of other symptoms well before the age of puberty, but occasionally growth failure and pubertal delay with minimal focal symptoms may be the presenting complaint. Self-imposed caloric restriction caused by an eating disorder such as anorexia nervosa presents most often with interrupted puberty or secondary amenorrhea, but it may be a cause of pubertal delay. A hypothalamic tumor should be excluded as a possible cause of poor food intake and delayed puberty in the prepubertal patient with an apparent eating disorder. Girls normally gain weight throughout childhood and adolescence. Even a small amount of weight loss or a failure to gain weight along a normal growth curve may represent significant nutritional compromise in a young teenager and warrants evaluation. Most young adolescent girls are very concerned about the possibility of being overweight. Some teenagers who do not have the complete picture of anorexia nervosa may actually interrupt their growth spurt and pubertal progression by overconcern about restricting their intake to a carefully controlled "healthy" diet low in fats and carbohydrates, which might be appropriate for an adult trying to reduce the risks of cardiovascular disease but that does not provide enough calories for growth.

Severe environmental stress may cause delayed puberty and growth failure in some individuals. As young female athletes have begun training intensively at earlier ages, delayed puberty caused by prolonged exercise has become more common. Delayed puberty occurs most commonly in sports such as ballet, gymnastics, and skating, which stress a lean body composition in addition to intensive training.

Endocrinopathies such as hypothyroidism or cortisol excess can present with slowing of statural growth and delayed puberty. The symptoms of acquired hypothyroidism can be quite subtle, and the disease is often present for a number of years before it is recognized. In contrast to the nutritional causes of delayed adolescence, weight is better preserved than height in an endocrinopathy such as hypothyroidism. Hypothyroid patients are usually moderately but not massively overweight for height. Patients with poorly controlled diabetes mellitus may have growth failure and delayed or interrupted puberty. The mechanism for this is unclear, but interference with reproductive function at the hypothalamic, pituitary, and ovarian levels have been described in diabetes.

HYPOTHALAMIC DYSFUNCTION

Local hypothalamic causes of delayed puberty in which puberty fails to proceed normally because of absence of pulsatile GnRH release include tumors, other mass lesions, hydrocephalus, and infiltrative lesions of the hypothalamus as well as congenital absence of GnRH production.

The most common tumor to present with delayed puberty and waning statural growth is a craniopharyngioma. Headaches and diabetes insipidus may be additional problems in some of these children. Gliomas and germinomas may also interfere with pubertal progression. Other mass lesions that may interrupt puberty are brain abscesses and granulomatous disease, such as tuberculosis or sarcoidosis.

Children who received central nervous system (CNS) irradiation for treatment of tumors or leukemia often sustain hypothalamic damage resulting in hypothalamic-pituitary hormonal insufficiencies that may emerge over a period of several years. Growth hormone deficiency is the most common; however, CNS irradiation may also damage GnRH release. These patients may have premature puberty, which then fades to failure of pubertal progression as late effects of radiation damage become evident. The hypothalamus is more sensitive to radiation damage than the pituitary.

Children who lack the ability to normally secrete GnRH may also have midline facial defects, such as cleft palate. Anosmia or hyposmia accompanying congenital lack of GnRH secretion is termed Kallman's syndrome. Kallman's syndrome is more common in males than in females, and it can be familial. Other syndromes that include hypothalamic hypogonadism are Prader–Willi syndrome (massive obesity and hyperphagia, short stature, small hands and feet, and mental retardation), and Lawrence–Moon–Biedl (retinitis pigmentosa, obesity, and extra digits).

Infiltrative lesions that may interrupt puberty include histiocytosis X, CNS leukemia, and hemochromatosis. Hemochromatosis is most commonly due to iron overload secondary to conditions that require repeated transfusions, such as thalassemia major. Dysfunction caused by iron overload may involve the pituitary, gonads, and end organ response to sex steroids as well.

PITUITARY DYSFUNCTION

Puberty may fail to occur if the pituitary cannot respond to GnRH signals with gonadotropin release. Hypopituitarism rarely follows head trauma or may occur either congenitally or in an acquired form with no obvious antecedent insult.

The most common pituitary tumor causing failure of pubertal progression in girls is a prolactinoma. Elevated prolactin levels interfere with GnRH secretion, and the tumors may also have mass effects compromising gonadotropin production in the pituitary. These tumors most commonly present in young adult women who develop secondary amenorrhea, galactorrhea, and headaches. In adolescents, prolactinomas may cause an interruption of pubertal progression. Galactorrhea is not present in all patients. One-half will have a history of galactorrhea, and in two-thirds, galactorrhea may be detected on exam. Headaches are frequent but not invariably present.

GONADAL DYSFUNCTION

Ovarian failure as a cause of delayed puberty is most commonly due to gonadal dysgenesis. The majority of these patients have gonadal dysgenesis on the basis of a chromosomal abnormality. Two X chromosomes are necessary for normal ovarian development. About half of the patients with gonadal dysgenesis have an XO blood karyotype. Most of the rest are mosaics or have a partial X chromosome deletion. The classic Turner's syndrome phenotype of webbed neck, low-set ears, widely spaced nipples, short fourth and fifth digits, and cubitus valgus is not always present. Short stature usually marked in XO gonadal dysgenesis with final height reaching an average of 56 inches without intervention. Mosaic patients may have less severe short stature. Some patients may have ovarian function that allows spontaneous puberty. Although ovarian function is usually short-lived, pregnancies can occur in these patients. Any patient with gonadal dysgenesis who has any evidence of androgen excess should be investigated for a Y cell line ("mixed gonadal dysgenesis") that can be limited to the gonad and predisposes the patient to develop gonadoblastomas and germ cell tumors. Therefore, these patients should have gonadectomies.

Pure gonadal dysgenesis occurs when the gonads fail to develop early in embryogenesis. Patients may be XX or XY by karyotype and have a normal prepubertal female phenotype without the stigmata of Turner's syndrome. Patients with XY gonadal dysgenesis may have a uterus if the gonad does not develop sufficiently to make Mullerian inhibiting factor. Patients with XY gonadal dysgenesis should have gonadectomies performed before they reach adulthood because of the risk of gonadal tumors.

Causes of ovarian failure with a normal karyotype include autoimmune oophoritis, which may present with interrupted puberty. These patients are at risk for other endocrinopathies, such as thyroiditis, diabetes mellitus, and Addison's disease as well as other autoimmune disease, and they should be followed. A family history of polyglandular endocrinopathy may be present. Ovarian damage by radiation or chemotherapy with alkylating agents may prevent puberty in survivors of childhood malignancies. Patients with galactosemia, sarcoidosis, myotonic dystrophy, or ataxia telangiectasia also can have ovarian failure.

Hypergonadotropic hypogonadism can also occur when the ovary cannot respond to gonadotropin stimulation with sex steroid synthesis. Inability to respond to the FSH stimulation has been termed the "resistant ovary syndrome" and may be transient in some patients. Very rarely, hypergonadotropic hypogonadism may be caused by defects in the enzyme pathways of sex steroid synthesis. A defect in cytochrome p450c17 (17 alpha hydroxylase) activity can block sex steroid production and present as sexual infantilism. A defect in 20-22 desmolase activity needed to convert cholesterol to pregnenolone may present similarly if the deficiency is primarily expressed in the gonads. These patients may be genetic males with an infantile female phenotype.

DELAYED MENARCHE

The young woman who has secondary sexual development but who does not have menarche within 4 years of starting breast development may have had an interruption of the pubertal process after its normal initiation. This may be due to a number of the central, hypothalamic, pituitary, or ovarian causes listed above. Alternatively, she may have an anatomic abnormality of the uterus or vagina preventing menstruation despite normal ovarian function. Anatomic abnormalities range from imperforate hymen to vaginal septum, cervical agenesis, or uterine agenesis, often with absence of the upper vagina as well (Rokitansky's syndrome). Patients who lack normal uterine development may have congenital malformations of the kidneys as well. Other congenital anomalies associated with abnormal formation of Mullerian duct structures include skeletal deformities such as Klippel–Feil syndrome.

An individual with an XY karyotype who has complete androgen insensitivity will have testes that secrete Mullerian inhibiting factor. Mullerian duct structures (the uterus and upper vagina), will therefore fail to develop. The testes are usually intraabdominal but may be noted as groin masses sometimes located during inguinal herniorrhaphy. These patients' testes make estradiol in addition to testosterone. Pituitary gonadotropins may be somewhat elevated, since testosterone does not feedback to suppress the pituitary gonadotropins. Testosterone is normal to increased for a male. The androgen resistance has been found to be due to either the absence of the testosterone receptor or the ability of the receptor-androgen complex to initiate androgen effects within target cells. Since these patients are normally sensitive to estradiol, they feminize at puberty with the development of breasts that are fully developed in appearance although less glandular than a normal female who has ductal proliferation under the influence of progesterone. Body hair and acne are decreased or absent. These patients are somewhat taller than average females and follow a height velocity curve that is appropriately timed for male puberty, although their final heights on average are intermediate between male and female.

A patient with androgen excess from an ovarian or adrenal source, most commonly "polycystic ovary syndrome" or mild congenital adrenal hyperplasia, may present with primary amenorrhea with secondary sexual development, although menarche at the normal time followed by oligomenorrhea is more common. These patients classically are obese and have physical evidence of androgen excess, such as hirsutism, acne, and sometimes slight clitoral enlargement. Hirsutism becomes more evident with time and may be minimal in the young adolescent. Evidence of insulin resistance, such as acanthosis nigricans, a muscular build, and thick digits, may be present in some patients with ovarian androgen excess.

EVALUATION OF THE PATIENT WITH DELAYED PUBERTY

Under the best of circumstances, adolescence is a tumultuous time when rapid growth and secondary sexual development require a young woman to acknowledge and accept herself as a changed person. Early adolescence is a time of great conformity where teenagers look to each other to reassure themselves that their physical appearance is similar to that of their contemporaries and that they are therefore normal. When a young woman's pattern of growth and development deviates from that of her classmates, her concept of herself as an intact, healthy person can be threatened severely. A consultation with a physician during this crisis is a highly emotionally charged event for the young teenager. A good experience can have a positive impact on her feelings about herself and her ability to constructively interact with health care providers in the future.

The physician need not be experienced in dealing with large numbers of adolescents to have a positive interaction with a teenager. All that is required is a recognition and respect for the patient as an individual distinct from her parents. As in all pediatric consultations, there are at least two concerned parties: the patient herself and her parents. Each will have separate issues and questions that they may be reluctant to voice in the presence of the other. It may be helpful to talk to the parents alone first both to review the medical history, and to give them a chance to discuss the impact of the problem on the patient's functioning in school, at home, and with peers. It is then useful to see the patient by herself. If time permits, it is helpful to meet the teenager, ask her concerns, and outline a general plan for the office visit before she undresses for her physical exam. During a review of systems, confidential questions about environmental stresses, sexual activity, and drug use may be asked. A simple explanation of the nature of the physical exam and any procedures or tests that the evaluation may entail is helpful in reducing her anxiety. The patient and her parents are likely to be worried about whether she will need a pelvic exam, and whether this would be physically traumatic to her. If a pelvic exam is needed, the patient and her parents can be told that the exam can be done easily and atraumatically, using techniques designed for the young adolescent, and that any procedures will be explained and will be done only with her cooperation. Following the physical exam, the parents and teenager can be invited back in to discuss impression and plan.

HISTORY AND PHYSICAL EXAM

A thorough history and physical exam can help to focus the evaluation and reduce the laboratory testing needed in the initial visit. The history is directed toward sorting out a functional delay of adolescence from the numerous organic problems at any of the points along the hypothalamic–pituitary–ovarian axis listed above. In contrast to boys, constitutional delay of puberty is rare in girls and is a diagnosis of exclusion.

Neonatal history should include any history of ingestion of hormones during gestation, previous maternal miscarriages, birth weight, any neonatal problems suggestive of hypopituitarism, such as hypoglycemia and history of congenital anomalies or neonatal edema (Turner's syndrome). Past medical history should include any history of chronic disease, surgery, radiation exposure, or chemotherapy.

Measurements of height and weight plotted on a growth chart are of special importance in evaluating any child with delayed puberty. The pattern of growth and any changes in that pattern are important clues that often lead to a diagnosis. If delayed puberty is due to poor nutrition caused by an eating disorder, inflammatory bowel disease or malabsorption, or chronic disease with increased energy requirements, there will be a greater fall off in weight gain than in height. The child whose pubertal delay is due to an endocrinopathy such as acquired hypothyroidism or cortisol excess will have weight gain better preserved than statural growth.

In review of systems, weight changes, dieting, stress, athletics, gastrointestinal symptoms, headaches, neurologic symptoms including loss of peripheral vision, and ability to smell are of special interest.

Family history should include the heights, timing of puberty, and history of gynecologic or reproductive dysfunction in family members. History of endocrinopathies, such as diabetes mellitus or thyroiditis, which might represent familial autoimmune polyglandular disease, should be sought.

The physical exam should include height, weight, and vital signs. The patient should be examined with special attention paid to any midline facial defects or congenital anomalies. Breast staging according to the method popularized by JM Tanner is useful assessing where an individual is in the pubertal process. Tanner B1 is no development, B2 is a nubin of tissue under the areola, B3 is a smooth mound of tissue extending well beyond the areola, B4 is a double contour of areola protruding beyond the surrounding breast tissue, and B5 is the adult smooth breast contour. In addition, it is helpful to measure the dimensions of areolae and glandular breast tissue as a bioassay of estrogen. Standards also exist for width of the papilla. If any breast development is present, an attempt should be made to express any milky discharge. The absence of galactorrhea does not exclude hyperprolactinemia.

The examination of the external genitalia should focus on a search for congenital anomalies, such as imperforate hymen and assessment of current estrogen effect. The vaginal mucosa will thicken and become pale pink under the influence of estrogen. Leukorrhea is another indication of estrogen effect, as is development of the labia minora. Tanner stages PH1–5 describe the progression of pubic hair development. Any evidence of androgen excess such as clitoromegaly or hirsutism should be noted.

A pelvic exam is not always necessary as a part of the initial visit in a girl with total absence of secondary sexual development, but it should be done to rule out congenital anomalies of the Mullerian structures in a patient who has normal pubertal development but delayed menarche. If the patient has hypergonadotropic hypogonadism, a pelvic exam may establish that a uterus is present. In most nonsexually active patients, the cervix can be visualized with the use of a Hoffman speculum. In the patient whose hymeneal opening is too small to admit a Hoffman speculum, a small saline-moistened swab can be used to establish that vaginal depth is normal. The uterus and adnexae can be assessed by bimanual rectoabdominal exam in the lithotomy position. Even in the patient who has had no estrogen exposure to stimulate the growth of the uterus, a cervix, if present, is usually palpable on rectoabdominal exam.

In the patient with delayed or interrupted puberty, neurologic exam should include visual fields by confrontation and olfactory testing.

LABORATORY TESTS

Initial laboratory studies may be focused by the diagnostic possibilities suggested by the history and physical exam. A bone age, a complete blood count with an erythrocyte sedimentation rate, LH, FSH, and estradiol or other assessment of estrogen effect are useful initial screening tests. Prolactin and thyroid function tests are often included.

A bone age is determined with the use of a radiograph of the left hand and wrist, which is compared to the Gruelich and Pyle or Tanner–Whitehouse standards for skeletal maturation. With the use of the Bayer and Bayley tables in the Gruelich and Pyle Atlas of Skeletal Maturation, a prediction of final adult height may be made. Although this is a rough estimate, it is useful in assessing the amount of statural growth remaining in the patient with short stature. Tables also exist for height prediction that uses the Tanner–Whitehouse system of assessing skeletal age. Delayed skeletal maturation may also be a clue to the diagnosis of an endocrinopathy; the patient who has acquired hypothyroidism will have a bone age that lags behind height age. Height age is defined as the age at which the patient's height would be at the fiftieth centile.

The complete blood count and erythrocyte sedimentation rate may point to a chronic illness, such as inflammatory bowel disease, underlying the failure of growth and pubertal development; however, a normal ESR does not exclude inflammatory bowel disease.

The pituitary gonadotropins LH and FSH are of special value in separating primary gonadal dysfunction from central causes of pubertal delay. If the LH and FSH are elevated, the patient has primary gonadal failure. A karyotype should be obtained in searching for a chromosomal abnormality resulting in gonadal dysgenesis. Newer DNA probe techniques can identify fragments of Y chromosome translocated to other chromosomes in some patients with gonadal dysgenesis previously thought to be simple 45 X. If the chromosomes are normal, antiovarian antibodies may be obtained looking for autoimmune oopheritis. A definitive diagnosis of autoimmune oopheritis versus the resistant ovary syndrome or 46 XX gonadal dysgenesis may have to await the results of an ovarian biopsy. Biopsy to document the presence or absence of follicles or lymphocytic infiltrate is usually postponed until the patient wishes definitive information about her fertility, often as a young adult.

A pelvic ultrasound is useful if the presence or configuration of the uterus or gonads cannot be assessed adequately by a pelvic exam.

Most patients with delayed puberty have normal prepubertal LH and FSH values. Daytime prepubertal gonadotropin values do not exclude pubertal activity, since these hormones may be secreted only in pulses during sleep in the early stages of puberty. A pubertal response of LH and FSH to a bolus of intravenous GnRH may be used to document activation of puberty, but it is seldom necessary.

If LH and FSH are in the normal prepubertal or pubertal range, further tests would then include prolactin and thyroid function tests. A cranial computed tomography scan or magnetic resonance imaging (MRI) scan can help to exclude CNS or pituitary tumors as a cause of delayed or interrupted puberty. A lateral skull radiograph may reveal hypothalamic calcification in the case of a craniopharyngioma or sellar erosion in the case of a prolactinoma, but it does not definitively rule out a tumor.

Breast growth and maturation of the vaginal mucosa and labia are more sensitive than a single daytime measurement of estradiol level as an indicator of ovarian activity. A maturation index or vaginal smear to assess estrogen effect quantitatively may be obtained by running a small, cotton-tipped swab along the vaginal wall from the depths of the vagina out toward the introitus and fixing it immediately using a fixative for Papanicolaou smear. A maturation index may also be obtained on a fresh spun urine specimen. With the use of Meisel's system of assigning one point for each superficial cell, and one-half point for each intermediate cell, a score of greater than 38 indicates definite estrogen effect.

If the patient has secondary sexual development with delayed menarche, medroxyprogesterone withdrawal may be used to induce a period. If there is a withdrawal bleed, adequate estrogen priming and a uterus must be present. If there is no withdrawal bleed, a cycle of estrogen and progestin may be used to determine that the anatomy permits a withdrawal bleed when adequate priming of the endometrium is provided. An adolescent may rarely be pregnant despite a history of primary amenorrhea; therefore, a pregnancy test should precede the use of medication to induce menses.

If the disruption of the pubertal process is due to a chronic disease or tumor, treatment is directed toward correction of that underlying condition. If it is not possible to correct the underlying problem, it may be necessary to induce puberty pharmacologically. The timing of induction of secondary sexual development should be such that final height is not unduly compromised. Prevention of osteopenia is another consideration in determination of when to induce puberty. Secondary sexual development is usually initiated by use of a low dose of estrogen in order to maximize statural growth.

The usual initial dose of conjugated equine estrogens (Premarin) is 0.3 mg per day by mouth. The patient's height and progression of development should be monitored at 3-month intervals, and the bone age followed at 6-month intervals. When growth slows, usually after 6 months to 1 year, the dose may be increased to 0.625 mg, and the patient is cycled with a progestin, such as medroxyprogesterone acetate, each month. Higher doses of estrogen are sometimes needed to induce regular menses. Controversy continues over the number of days of estrogen and progestin required for optimal prevention of osteopenia and endometrial hyperplasia. Twenty-five days of estrogen each month with 12 days of progestin (days 14–25) is one commonly used regimen.

Estradiol dermal patches are a recent development for maintaining estrogen effect that some adolescents find acceptable. If the patient has absent or interrupted puberty caused by hypogonadotropic hypogonadism on a hypothalamic basis, pulsatile GnRH given intravenously or subcutaneously by pump may be used to initiate ovarian function. This is most often used at the time when fertility is desired. Donor egg implantation offers new possibilities for pregnancy in patients with gonadal dysgenesis or ovarian failure who have a normal uterus. Trials of using human growth hormone with or without oxandrolone to improve final height in patients with Turner's syndrome are now in progress with encouraging early results. Like all studies of interventions to improve growth, these studies will have to be continued until patients reach their final adult height before the benefit of this approach can be determined.

Patients who have a permanent defect in reproductive function can benefit greatly from ongoing counseling and support from a health care provider throughout their adolescence. Efforts should be made to help these teenagers develop concepts of themselves as capable, emerging adults. Often it is necessary to review the nature of their particular physiology a number of times and to explore gently their understanding of their situation as they return for follow-up visits. Emphasis should be placed on the patient's ability to function normally as an adult, perhaps with the help of hormonal replacement. Questions about fertility are best handled at the time they are brought up by the patient. Technological advances continue to open new doors to infertile patients, so that infertility may not be absolute. Patients may often be reluctant to share their fears that they will not be able to function as a sexual or marriage partner. They can be reassured that they can expect to be a successful marriage partner and a parent to adopted children.

BIBLIOGRAPHY

Chapman AJ: Delayed Puberty. Br Med J 1985;290:1493.
Ojeda SR, Andrews WW, Advis JP, et al: Recent advances in the endocrinology of puberty. Endocr Rev 1980;1:228.

Reindollar RH, Byrd JR, McDonough PG: Delayed sexual development: A study of 252 patients. Am J Obstet Gynecol 1981;140:371.

Reindollar RH, McDonough PG: Pubertal abberancy. Etiology and clinical approach. J Reprod Med 1984;29:391.

Reiter EO, Grumbach MM: Neuroendocrine control mechanisms and the onset of puberty. Ann Rev Physiol 1982;44:595.

Root AW: Hormonal changes in puberty. Pediatric Ann 1980;9:365.

Styne DM, Grumbach MM: Puberty in the male and female: its physiology and disorders. In: Yen SSC, Jaffe RB, eds. *Reproductive endocrinology,* 2nd ed. Philadelphia, WB Saunders Co, 1986.

Apter D, Viinikka L, Vihko R: Hormonal pattern of adolescent menstrual cycles. J Clin Endocrinol Metab 1978;47:944.

Belchetz PE, Plant TM, Lakai Y, et al: Hypophyseal responses to continuous and intermittent delivery of hypothalamic gonadotropin-releasing hormone. Science 1978;202:631.

Boyer RM, Finkelstein JW, David R, et al: Synchronization of augmented luteinizing hormone secretion with sleep during puberty. N Engl J Med 1972;287:582.

Boyer RM, Finkelstein JW, David R, et al: Simultaneous augmented secretion of luteinizing hormone and testosterone during sleep. J Clin Invest 1974;54:609.

Conte FA, Grumbach MM, Kaplan SL, et al: Correlation of luteinizing hormone-releasing factor-induced luteinizing hormone and follicle stimulating hormone release from infancy to 19 years with the changing pattern of gonadotropin secretion in agonadal patients: relation to the restraint of puberty. J Clin Endocrinol Metab 1980;50:163.

Filicori M, Santoro N, Merriam GR, et al: Characterization of the physiological pattern of episodic gonadotropin secretion throughout the human menstrual cycle. J Clin Endocrinol Metab 1986;62:1136.

Jakacki RI, Kelch RP, Sauder SE, et al: Pulsatile secretion of luteinizing hormone in children. J Clin Endocrinol Metab 1982;55:453.

Kaplan SL, Grumbach MM, Aubert ML: The ontogenesis of pituitary hormones and hypothalamic factors in the human fetus. Maturation of central nervous system regulation of anterior pituitary function. Recent Prog Horm Res 1976;34:161.

Lemarchand-Beraud T, Zufferey MM, Reymond M, et al: Maturation of the hypothalamo-pituitary-ovarian axis in adolescent girls. J Clin Endocrinol Metab 1982;54:241.

Lucky AW, Rich BH, Rosenfield RL, et al: LH bioactivity increases more than immunoreactivity during puberty. J Pediatr 1980;97:205.

Petraglia F, Bernasconi S, Iughetti L, et al: Naloxone-induced luteinizing hormone secretion in normal, precocious, and delayed puberty. J Clin Endocrinol Metab 1986;63:1112.

Reiter EO, Beitins IZ, Ostrea T, et al: Bioassayable luteinizing hormone during childhood and adolescence and in patients with delayed pubertal development. J Clin Endocrinol Metab 1982;54:155.

Ross JL, Loriaux DL, Cutler GB: Developmental changes in neuroendocrine regulation of gonadotropin secretion in gonadal dysgenesis. J Clin Endocrinol Metab 1983;57:288.

Talbert LM, Hammond MG, Groffe T, et al: Relationship of age and pubertal development to ovulation in adolescent girls. Obstet Gynecol 1985;66:542.

Waldhauser F, Weibenbacher G, Frisch H, et al: Pulsatile secretion of gonadotropins in early infancy. Eur J Pediatr 1981;137:71.

Waldhauser F, Weiszenbacher G, Frisch H, et al: Fall in nocturnal serum melatonin during prepuberty and pubescence. Lancet 1984;II:632.

Winter JSD, Faiman C, Hobson WC, et al: Pituitary gonadal relations in infancy. I. Patterns of serum gonadotropin concentration from birth to four years of age in man and chimpanzee. J Clin Endocrinol Metab 1975;40:545.

Copeland KC, Paunier L, Sizonenko PC: The secretion of adrenal androgens and growth patterns of patients with hypogonadotropic hypogonadism and idiopathic delayed puberty. J Pediatr 91:985.

Cutler GB, Loriaux DL: Adrenarche and its relationship to the onset of puberty. Fed Proc 1980;39:2384.

Dhom G: The prepubertal and pubertal growth of the adrenal (adrenarche). Beitr Path Bd 1973;150:357.

Ilondo MM, Vanderschueren-Lodeweyckx M, Vlietinck R, et al: Plasma androgens in children and adolescents. Part I. Control subjects. Hormone Res 1982;16:61.

Reiter EO, Fuldauer VG, Root AW: Secretion of the adrenal androgen dehydroepiandrosterone sulfate, during normal infancy, childhood, and adolescence, in sick infants, and in children with endocrinologic abnormalities. J Pediatr 1977;90:766.

Rich BH, Rosenfield RL, Lucky AW, et al: Adrenarche: changing adrenal response to adrenocotricotropin. J Clin Endocrinol Metab 1981;52:1129.

Scheibinger RJ, Albertson BD, Cassorla FG, et al: The developmental changes in plasma adrenal androgens during infancy and adrenarche are associated with changing activities of adrenal microsomal 17-hydroxylase and 17,20 desmolase. J Clin Invest 1981;67:1177.

Sizonenko PC, Paunier L, Carmignac D: Hormonal changes during puberty. IV. longitudinal study of adrenal androgen secretions. Horm Res 1976;7:288.

Korth-Schutz S, Levine LS, New MI: Serum androgens in normal prepubertal and pubertal children and in children with precocious adrenarche. J Clin Endocrinol Metab 1976;42:117.

Sklar CA, Kaplan SL, Grumbach MM: Evidence for dissociation between adrenarche and gonadarche: studies in patients with idiopathic precocious puberty, gonadal dysgenesis, isolated gonadotropin deficiency, and constitutionally delayed growth and adolescence. J Clin Endocrinol Metab 1980;51:548.

Harlan WR, Harlan EA, Grillo GP: Secondary sex characteristics of girls 12 to 17 years of age: The U.S. Health examination survey. J Pediatr 1980;96:1074.

Marshall WA, Tanner JM: Variations in the pattern of pubertal changes in girls. Arch Dis Child 1969;44:291.

Nottelman ED, Susman EJ, Inoff-Germain G, et al: Developmental processes in early adolescence: relationships between adolescent adjustment problems and chronologic age, pubertal stage, and puberty-related serum hormone levels. J Pediatr 1987;110:473.

Rohn RD: Nipple (papilla) development in puberty: longitudinal observations in girls. Pediatrics 1987;79:745.

Stanhope R, Adams J, Jacobs HS, et al: Ovarian ultrasound assessment in normal children, idiopathic precocious puberty, and during low dose pulsatile gonadotrophin releasing hormone treatment of hypogonadotropic hypogonadism. Arch Dis Child 1985;60:116.

Tanner JM, Whitehouse RH, Takaishi M: Standards from birth to maturity for height, weight, height velocity and weight velocity: British children, 1965. Part 2. Arch Dis Child 1966;41:613.

Tanner JM, Davies PSW: Clinical longitudinal standards for height and height velocity for North American children. J Pediatr 1985;107:317.

Wyshak G, Frisch RE: Evidence for a secular trend in age of menarche. N Engl J Med 1982;306:1033.

Frish RE, McArthur JW: Menstrual cycles: Fatness as a determinant of minimum weight for height necessary for their maintenance or onset. Science 1974;185:949.

Galler JR, Ramsey F, Solimano G: A follow-up study of early malnutrition on subsequent development. 1. Physical growth and sexual maturation during adolescence. Pediatr Res 1985;19:518.

Kulin HE, Bwibo N, Mutie D, et al: The effect of chronic malnutrition on pubertal growth and development. Am J Clin Nutr 1982;36:527.

Kulin HE, Bwibo N, Mutie D, et al: Gonadotropin excretion during puberty in malnourished children. J Pediatr 1984;105:325.

Pugliese MT, Lifshitz F, Grad G, et al: Fear of obesity. A cause of short stature and delayed puberty. N Engl J Med 1983;309:513.

Schwartz B, Cumming DC, Riofdan E, et al: Exercise-associated amenorrhea: a distinct entity? Am J Obstet Gynecol 1981;141:662.

Warren MP: The effects of exercise on pubertal progression and reproductive function in girls. J Clin Endocrinol Metab 1980;51:1150.

Warren MP: Effects of undernutrition on reproductive function in the human. Endocr Rev 1983;4:363.

Warren MP, Brooks-Gunn J, Hamilton LH, et al: Scoliosis and fractures in young ballet dancers. N Engl J Med 1986;314:1348.

Kauli R, Schoenfeld A, Ovadia Y, et al: Delayed puberty and hypoplastic uterus associated with hyperprolactinemia: successful treatment with bromocryptine. Horm Res 1985;22:68.

Sack J, Friedman E, Tadmor R, et al: Growth and puberty arrest due to prolactinoma. Acta Paediatr Scand 1984;73:863.

Rivkees SA, Bode HH, Crawford JD: Long-term growth in juvenile acquired hypothyroidism: the failure to achieve normal adult stature. N Engl J Med 1988;318:599.

Fisher DA: Catch-up growth in hypothyroidism. N Engl J Med 1988;318:632.

Page DC, Mosher R, Simpson EM, et al: The sex-determining region of the hyman Y chromosome encodes a finger protein. Cell 1987;51:1091.

Magenis RE, Tochen ML, Holahan KP, et al: Turner syndrome resulting from partial deletion of Y chromosome short arm: localization of male determinants. J Pediatr 1984;105:916.

Brook CGD: Management of delayed puberty. Br Med J 1985;290:657.

Chetkowsi RJ, Meldrum DR, Steingold KA, et al: Biologic effects of transdermal estradiol. N Engl J Med 1986;314:1615.

Rosenfield RL, Furlanetto: Physiologic testosterone or estradiol induction of puberty increases plasma somatomedin-C. Am J Dis Child 1985;107:415.

Wagner TOF, Brabant G, Warsch R, et al: Pulsatile gonadotropin-releasing hormone treatment in idiopathic delayed puberty. J Clin Endocrinol Metab 1986;62:95.

CHAPTER 3

Sexual Abuse in the Pediatric and Adolescent Patient

Marietta Murphy, MD

Sexual molestation is a problem exploding into epidemic proportions. Given its high prevalence and occurrence in all ethnic and social classes, it appears to be a problem that will not just go away. The most conservative retrospective surveys of adults based on episodes of actual contact reveal 1 in 5 girls and 1 in 10 boys as sexually abused.[1] In 1981, the National Center on Child Abuse and Neglect reported 45,000 cases of confirmed sexual abuse involving a parent or caretaker every year. No numbers are available from them on assaults by others. In general, authorities estimate that only 10% of cases are reported, leaving us with an estimate of a child being sexually abused or molested at least once every 2 minutes somewhere in the United States.[2]

DEFINITIONS

Legal definitions vary from state to state but are in a state of flux as the criminal justice system struggles to respond to demands by clinicians and children for protection from assaults that may not readily yield corroborative evidence. Clinically, though, we must deal with sexual assault from the perspective that cases that may not be proven legally may have lifelong impact on an individual child's reproductive capacity both physically and psychologically. Sexually transmitted diseases are becoming increasingly prevalent in children under 15, particularly prepubertal children.

Lacerations and other genital trauma, while not necessarily correlated with chronic sexual abuse, leave lasting scars. We see other short-term problems, such as depression, phobic reaction, and somaticization, as well as long-term problems related to drug abuse,[3] juvenile delinquency,[4] pros-

Clinical Practice of Gynecology: 3, 31–39, 1989
© 1989 Elsevier Science Publishing Co., Inc.
655 Avenue of the Americas, New York, NY 10010

ISSN 1043-3198/89/$3.50

titution,[5] and adult depression.[6] One can only speculate how this may be related to the enormous problem of infertility.

Underscoring the tremendous clinical impact of sexual abuse, we use the definitions developed by the Children's Hospital National Medical Center, Washington, DC, as any situation involving any one or more of the following activities:

- Sexual assault involving physical force in which a child is the victim.
- Sexual contact or interaction between a child and another person of any age in which the child's participation has been obtained through undue means, such as threats, bribery, or coercion.
- Sexual contact or interaction between a child and an adult or other person, even with the free cooperation of the child, when such activity is inappropriate to the age and level of maturity of the other person.[7]

SPECTRUM

These definitions yield a spectrum of assault with a high level of morbidity. They also reveal a range of child molestation that appears to follow a progressive pattern. This pattern has been outlined in the *Handbook of Clinical Intervention in Child Sexual Abuse*[8] as progressing from exposure to fondling, mutual masturbation to actual intercourse. In a 3-year study at Children's Hospital National Medical Center, the most common types of sexual abuse seen were vaginal intercourse (41.7%), anal intercourse (20.3%), fondling (18.2%), fellatio (13.8%), and manual vaginal intercourse (10%). The methods used to engage children were physical force, most often physical restraint (49.7%), threat of bodily harm (40.4%), the child's duty to obey adult authority (19.2%), bribery (16.9%), and misrepresentations of standards (15.2%).[9] An ongoing analysis at The Children's Hospital, Boston, reveals similar patterns of assault.

Who is being assaulted and by whom? As stated previously, there is no predominant pattern of victims or offenders with respect to social class or ethnic background. Ages of children seen at The Children's Hospital, Boston, range from 8 months to 19 years with a peak between 6 and 9 years. Fifteen percent of the victims at The Children's Hospital, Boston, are boys, with other centers reporting from 5% to 25%. Violent assault and sexually transmitted disease tend to cluster at either end of the age range but are seen throughout. Similar distributions are observed at other major centers.

The pattern that is identifiable refers to the offenders. Children are not being molested by pedophilic strangers. Molestation overwhelmingly is perpetrated by people well known to the child—parent figures (25%), other family members (17%), or friends of the family (38%), who may well be maintaining heterosexual relationships. Only 15–20% of reported assaults are by strangers. Perpetrators are predominantly male (95%), and an increasing proportion are under age 17 (35%). At least one-third of the perpetrators lived with the victim, and 46% of the abuse was repetitive. Parents are the most likely to engage in repetitive abuse (75%) as well as physically harm the child, but 62% of the parental figure offenders are not the biologic parent.[10]

APPROACH

Given this pattern of molestation, what should be our approach to victims? These children and families present a complex array of problems on presentation, and in order to impact on this damaging situation and effectively intervene on behalf of the child, we must approach it not only from the medical point of view but also from the psychologic and protective. A team approach with the Departments of Medicine, Social Services, and Psychiatry each evaluating and formulating a treatment plan for the family is currently felt to be the most effective standard of care. Each child needs protection either within the family or elsewhere, if the family cannot or will not do it. Each child will need help with short-term psychologic reactions and, for some, long-term sequelae. All of the children need complete medical evaluations both to reassure them that they are normal as well as to address the more common medical sequelae of sexually transmitted diseases and pregnancy.

SEXUALLY TRANSMITTED DISEASES

The most common sexually transmitted disease (STD) encountered in evaluating sexually abused children is gonorrhea. According to the Centers for Disease Control (CDC), the incidence, generally, in prepubertal children aged 0–14 years is 17.7/10,000.[11] Reviews have documented rates in sexually abused children ranging from 6% to 13%.[12] Gonorrhea in children 1–10 years of age was found to be transmitted sexually in 98% of cases in a study by Branch and Paxton.[13] Given the necessity of mucosal surface contact for the transmission of this fastidious organism, even in children, the finding of gonorrhea places sexual abuse high in the differential. Other STDs are also seen. Syphilis, while seemingly less prevalent, is worrisome because children rarely have clinical features. Although most children with syphilis will have another STD, for some if we don't look for it, we won't find it.

Condyloma acuminata, a growth caused by papilloma virus, has been well documented as sexually transmitted and raises the specter of sexual abuse when it presents in children beyond the age of 20 months, when it could have been transmitted intrapartum.[14] Trichomonas, as an STD in childhood, has not been well studied but is clearly transmitted through intimate contact that would be considered inappropriate for a child.[15] Herpes simplex type 2 is being seen increasingly in children, giving rise to the need to

Table 3-1. Sexually Transmitted Disease Pathogens

Bacteria
   Neisseria gonorrhea
   Treponema pallidum
   Hemophilus vaginalis
   Campylobacter fetus
   Shigella species
Others
   Chlamydia trachomatis
   Mycoplasma hominis
   Ureaplasma urealyticum
Viruses
   Condyloma acuminata (papilloma virus)
   Herpes simplex
   Hepatitis A & B
Protozoa
   Trichomonas vaginalis
   Entamoeba histolytica
   Giardia lamblia
Fungi
   Candida albicans

investigate sexual contact.[16] *Chlamydia trachomatis* is the most prevalent sexually transmitted disease in adults, but its diagnosis, as a result of sexual misuse, is difficult because of the need for cell culture technique or serologic testing, which can be confusing in children. Its long latency period (up to several years) and asymptomatic carriage add to its potential as a pathogen for sexually abused children, although two recent studies showed lower frequencies from 4% to 6%[17,18] (Table 3-1).

PREGNANCY

Pregnancy in any adolescent is generally considered high risk. From a maternal point of view, it not only disrupts normal adolescent development and attainment of educational goals but also exposes the adolescents to a higher risk of maternal morbidity, specifically from toxemia. From the child's perspective, higher perinatal morbidity and mortality, which increases with the birth order during the mother's adolescence, would have significant impact. In addition, the diagnosis is often made later in the pregnancy, complicating it by inadequate prenatal care. Preliminary data from The Children's Hospital, Boston, showed that of 90 at-risk adolescents, 9 became pregnant as a result of an alleged assault or incestuous relationship, and only 1 was diagnosed on initial evaluation.

MEDICAL EVALUATION

Given both the general and specific medical concerns, the approach to the child who presents with a complaint of alleged sexual abuse or in whom there are signs or symptoms that could be referable to sexual abuse must include an assessment of the entire child. A complete pediatric history, including specific questioning about prior genital infections, urinary complaints, toileting, developmental issues, and behavioral symptoms, in addition to the specifics of the alleged incident(s) in the patient's words, is required to begin to establish a data base. Adolescents need a thorough gynecologic history, including prior examinations and their purpose, as well as tampon usage, as these may influence the interpretation of findings, especially in younger adolescents. A general physical examination should always be performed despite the localized nature of the assault by history. Too often, children will not or may not have the vocabulary to divulge the true scope of the assault. In addition, other indications of neglect may be found on physical examinations. Specimens needed for collection are outlined in Table 3-2. In general, the pelvic evaluation should be incorporated within the context of the general physical exam and preferably in the same room in order to avoid undue focus on the genitalia or further trauma to the patient.

Children can be examined in a developmental manner, adapting the traditional gynecologic approach to their very different anatomic state (Table 3-3). Throughout the entire exam, each step should be explained either verbally or through doll play or drawings, and the child reassured and in control before proceeding. Prepubertal girls are examined in a knee–chest position to inspect their genitalia. Their short, hypoestrogenized vaginas are easily visualized, usually to the cervix in this position without speculae.[19] There is some evidence that measuring the hymenal opening in a relaxed child in the frog leg position may be helpful. A measurement of greater than 4 mm has been correlated with sexual abuse in a study by Kantwell.[20]

Specimens are collected using soft Clinitest droppers or moistened nasopharyngeal swabs in this position or supine in a frog-legged or lithotomy position. Palpation is performed using a rectoabdominal bimanual technique. Peripubertal girls may need a variety of approaches to examine their genitalia. Depending on their anatomy, knee–chest position may be used to visualize their vaginas. Some girls may be able to cooperate with a speculum exam, generally using the narrow Huffman speculum. Collection of specimens may be difficult in this age group, and careful, supervised self-sampling or participation by holding the labia often helps the child cooperate. A careful rectoabdominal bimanual exam will often answer questions, such as those about foreign body placement, or allow the examiner to milk out small amounts of vaginal discharge or blood that cannot be seen.

Postpubertal young women can generally cooperate with speculum

Table 3-2. Specimens for Collection

Clothing	If involved in alleged assault, should be placed in paper bag (not plastic), labeled and handed to police
Skin	Wood's lamp examination of skin may reveal fluorescent (dark green or blue green) areas; sample with moistened Q-tip, label, include with rape kit; screening test tape for acid phosphatase may also be used
Fingernails	Scrape under fingernails and enclose in envelope in rape kit
Throat	Culture for gonorrhea
Pubic hair	Comb for stray hairs; place in envelope in rape kit; a pubic hair from the victim should be enclosed in the standard envelope for comparison
Perineum	Wipe with 2 × 2 gauze pads moistened with distilled water and test for acid phosphatase with test tape enclosed in rape kit; if positive (positive is a deep purple color change immediately), enclose tape and both gauze pads in rape kit for analysis
Vaginal secretions	Slides Wet mount for sperm, trichomonads, cells KOH for yeast Gram stain for cells, flora Two (2) air dried slides for rape kit (sperm and acid phosphatase stain) Culture for gonorrhea Vaginal pool—prepubertally Cervical—postpubertally Papanicolaou smear Sperm, trichomonads, cells
Rectum	Culture for gonorrhea
Blood	RPR or VDRL Pregnancy test (if urine negative and clinically appropriate) Blood type (if evidence submitted may yield the blood group antigen of the assailant)
Urine	Urinalysis (cells, trichomonads, cells) Culture (if appropriate) Pregnancy test

exams by using the narrow Huffman type especially when there is trauma or swelling. Careful vaginal, abdominal, or rectoabdominal bimanuals yield similar information.

Recently, colposcopic examination has begun to be used in the evaluation of victims of sexual assault. Based on a forensic study from Brazil,[21] a group at Los Angeles Children's Hospital and The Children's Hospital, Boston, are beginning to study the use of the colposcopy in children who have been sexually molested.

Table 3-3.

	Approximate Age		
	8 Years Old	**8–11 Years Old**	**12 Years Old**
Visualization	Knee/chest position with otoscope light (no speculum required)*	Knee/chest or lithotomy, depending on anatomy and comfort	Lithotomy position with narrow vaginal speculum (Huffman or Pederson)
Collection of specimens	Aspirate with soft dropper; NP swab	Aspirate with soft dropper; NP swab	Moistened cotton-tipped swab
Palpation	Rectoabdominal bimanual exam	Rectoabdominal or one-finger vaginal exam	Vaginal–abdominal bimanual exam with one or two fingers

*If the prepubertal female is relaxed, her degree of lordosis will increase, and her abdomen will "sag" toward table. In this position, there is usually good visualization of the vagina and cervix.

The use of a rape kit during the initial examination is critical to increase the yield of corroborative evidence and to avoid repetitive exams. Rape kits are merely standardized means of collecting materials so that they can be used as evidence. Opening a rape kit does not imply that you must go to court but, in fact, may save the child further exposure. The contents of the rape kit used at The Children's Hospital, Boston, include envelopes for fingernail scrapings and pubic hair combings, in addition to a comb, a test tape for acid phosphatase with 2×2 gauze pads, two slides in a holder, a Papanicolaou smear spatula, and evidence stickers. The chain of evidence is preserved by either handing the enclosed rape kit to a detective or police officer by the examining doctor or nurse if the assault was reported to the police, or locking it in a safe and documenting the date, time, and person in a log.

At The Children's Hospital, Boston, we have developed a protocol approach for the emergency evaluation of children presenting with alleged sexual abuse or with symptoms or signs referable to it. Each child undergoes a complete medical examination using the rape kit to collect possible evidence. The family is evaluated by Social Services to determine the protective needs of the child and the family's ability to provide for those needs. A psychiatrist evaluates all children under 15 and adolescents experiencing severe crisis reactions. This is particularly important for younger children, as often the history begins to unfold in a different manner when one is using child psychiatric interviewing techniques.

Medical treatment on initial evaluation is directed toward prophylaxis of both venereal disease and pregnancy. If an infection is not detected on exam, prophylaxis against gonorrhea contact can be given with amoxicillin 3.0 gm or 50 mg/kg and probenecid 1 gm or 20 mg/kg. Broader prophylaxis against gonorrhea infection and incubating syphilis is provided with procaine penicillin 4.8 million U or 100,000 U/kg in two divided doses and Probenecid.

Pregnancy prophylaxis can be offered if coitus has occurred within the prior 72 hours, and the patient is not already pregnant. Diethylstilbestrol or Premarin 15–25 mg twice a day for 5 days can be used, but nausea and vomiting often compromise compliance. At The Children's Hospital, Boston, we are using Ovral, 2 mg, 2 tablets in the emergency room and 2 tablets, 12 hours later with good results since overall compliance is higher.

Medical, psychiatric, and social service follow-up are arranged in the emergency room before the family leaves. In a review from The Children's Hospital, Boston, medical follow-up at 1 week and 6 weeks have yielded concerning rates or morbidity. Venereal disease was diagnosed or treated in 22% of cases. Adolescents had particularly high rates of subsequent morbidity from pelvic inflammatory disease (PID) (10%) and pregnancy (19%). Behavioral disorders were uncovered in 23% of patients. Clearly, this is a population in need of aggressive outreach and services to address their significant risk for serious sequelae.

REFERENCES

1. Finkelhor D: Sexually victimized children. New York: The Free Press, 1979.
2. National Center of Child Abuse and Neglect. Study findings: National study of the severity of child abuse and neglect. Washington, DC: U.S. Government Printing Office, DHHS Publ No (OHDS) 81-30325, 1981.
3. Benward J, Densen-Gerber J: Incest as a causative factor in antisocial behavior: An exploratory study. Contemp Drug Prob 1975;332.
4. Halleck SL: The physician's role in management of victims of sex offenders. JAMA 1962;180:273.
5. James J, Meyerding J: Early sexual experience and prostitution. Am J Psychiatry 1977;134:1381.
6. Summit R, Kryso J: Sexual abuse of children: A clinical spectrum. Am J Ortho-Psychiatry 1978;48:237.
7. Clinical proceedings: Children's Hospital National Medical Center 40/3&4, 213.
8. Sgroi S: Handbook of clinical intervention in child sexual abuse. Lexington Books. 1982;12.
9. Data from Children's Hospital National Medical Center, Washington, DC: Division of Child Protection and The Children's Hospital, Boston, Emergency Services.
10. Clinical proceedings: Children's Hospital National Medical Center, 40/3&4, 215–217.
11. Morbidity and Mortality Weekly Report, annual summary, 1980: U.S. DHHS, MMWR 1981;29:38.
12. White S: Sexually transmitted diseases in sexually abused children. Pediatrics 1983;72.
13. Branch G, Paxton R: A study of gonococcal infections among infants and children. Public Health Rep 1965;80:347–352.
14. Seidel: Condyloma acuminata as a sign of sexual abuse in children. J Pediatr 1979;95:553–554.
15. DeJong AR: Condyloma acuminata in children. Am J Dis Child 1982;136:704–706.
16. Jaffe AC: Sexual abuse and herpetic genital infection in children (letter). J Pediatr 1976;89:338.

17. Ingram DL, et al: Vaginal chlamydial trachomatis infection in children with sexual contact. Pediatr Infect Dis 1984;3:97–99.
18. Hammerschlag MR, et al: Are recto-vaginal chlamydial infections a marker of sexual abuse in children. Pediatr Infect Dis 1984;3:100–104.
19. Emans SJ, Goldstein DP: Pediatric and adolescent gynecology, 2nd ed. Boston: Little, Brown, 1983.
20. Kantwell H: Vaginal inspection and child sexual abuse. Child Abuse Negl 1983;7:171–176.
21. Goncalves Treixeira WR: Hymenal colposcopic examination in sexual offenses. Am J Forensic Med Pathol 1981;2:209–214.

CHAPTER 4

Contraception

Maureen M. Lynch, MD

Contraceptive choices for the adolescent are unfortunately neither freer of human or method failure nor more appealing to the adolescent than they are for the more responsible patient. The special considerations stem from the patient's adolescence. Whether or not a physician ethically endorses premarital sexual relations, the fact remains that adolescents are engaging in intercourse at earlier ages—many, unfortunately, without the benefit of contraception. In their surveys of sexual behavior, Zelnick and Kantner[1] found that reported sexual activity among 15–19-year-old adolescents increased from 30% in 1971 to 50% in 1979. Of the sexually active in this group, only 34% always used contraception, 39% sometimes did, and 27% never used contraception. These frightening statistics obviously challenge each of us. The primary physician's role in managing sexually active adolescents is to enable them to make informed decisions about the degrees of intimacy and sexual involvement for which they are ready and can assume responsibility.

Because a teenager 14 or 15 years old will rarely seek out a discussion about contraception explicitly, the physician must incorporate the sexual history and the need for birth control into the routine history and physical. The teenager must be made to feel comfortable and secure and should not be interrogated or judged by the medical personnel. The woman college student, on the other hand, will seek gynecologic care on her own and, therefore, will receive anticipatory contraceptive counseling.

The degree of experience with and knowledge of contraception on the part of the primary care doctor will determine if the younger female patient needs to be referred to an obstetrician-gynecologist. In the course of training, one ought to have become adept in giving routine gynecologic care to

Clinical Practice of Gynecology: **3,** 40–51, 1989
© 1989 Elsevier Science Publishing Co., Inc.
655 Avenue of the Americas, New York, NY 10010

Table 4-1.

Contraception	Pregnancy Rates/ 100 Woman-Yrs. of Use
Comb. pill	0.1 – 0.7
CU7	1.0 – 2.5
Mini-pill	1.5 – 3.0
Diaphragm or Condom	3.0 – 20
Cervical cap	8
Contraceptive foam	3.0 – 30

an adolescent. It is also necessary to be well informed about the methods of birth control, their availability, and their indications and contraindications. The primary care physician must also be aware of the efficacy and side effects of the various methods, in case the patient has a specific problem. If the physician chooses to refer the patient, it is important to ascertain whether the new physician will deal with the adolescent patient in a sensitive, confidential, and nonjudgmental manner. Health care personnel dealing with a minor over such sensitive and charged issues as abortion and birth control need to keep in mind a number of issues that do not arise with the adult patient. Adolescents have their own legal status and legal rights. Therefore, it is our responsibility as medical providers to acquaint ourselves with the laws of the individual states. We must also remain aware of social factors influencing the prescribing of birth control to minors, ie, community, religious, and family constraints. Finally, counseling an adolescent must be conducted in meaningful terms. For example, it makes little sense to talk to a very young adolescent about the desirability of finishing college if she is barely finishing high school. One must also be willing and able to spend a good deal of time going through what future plans are realistic for the particular person. One must explore the implications of sexual activity and the responsibility of both partners concerning pregnancy and the occurrence of sexually transmitted diseases. In the course of this discussion about birth control, the most important information a caretaker can give the adolescent is that the risk of pregnancy to her life, health, and social well-being is far greater than the risk of any birth control method. One must also do serious counseling about AIDS control and safer sex practices.[2]

The actual pregnancy rates for 100 women using different contraceptive methods for 1 year (100 woman-years of use) are listed in Table 4-1. For example, the success of the method for the combination pill is 99.3–99.7% effective, for the diaphragm 80–97% effective, and so on. However, frequently the effectiveness of the method may be lower in the younger adolescent because of decreased compliance. (Compliance has been shown to be greater in a patient who is older, lives in a suburban neighborhood, has married parents, and is not on some form of public assistance for payment of medical bills.[3] In order to increase success rates for all adolescents, we should continue to encourage contraceptive education and school-based clinics, especially for high-risk patients.[4]

The anticipatory guidance should be tailored for the individual patient. Written instructions, which seem to get misplaced by the adolescent, should be supplemented with careful verbal instructions that seek to answer the teen's questions as thoroughly as possible. The more the teenager feels that she has participated in the visit and in the choice of the contraceptive method, the greater the chance that she will return for a follow-up visit and that she will comply with the physician's instructions. Identification of the noncompliant patient in advance and seeing that patient more frequently can be a worthwhile exercise for all concerned. When beginning to counsel an adolescent who is contemplating the responsibility of a mature and intimate sexual relationship, we need to be very careful to support the teenager's role in making her decision. Although we cannot be naive, we do not need to be yet another pressure on the teenager to be sexually active by assuming that she is asking for contraception when she appears for a gynecologic problem. It is very important to make it clear that the choice of abstinence is still a viable one.

If the choice to become sexually active is made, we need to determine with the teenager what her immediate needs for birth control are and what frequency she expects in her sexual relationship. In prescribing birth control, we also need to take into account any pertinent medical or gynecologic problems that the patient may have. For example, if the patient needs birth control and suffers from severe dysmenorrhea and/or hypermenorrhea, then she may do very well on the pill—provided that there are no contraindications. The patient also needs to understand that there is always an opportunity to change methods of birth control and that starting on one method does not require her to stay on it for her entire reproductive life. We also need to dispel any false information that the teenager has received from either her peers or parents about risks of contraception. Although the mortality rate in young, sexually active women is slightly lower for the barrier forms of contraception when coupled with optional use of a therapeutic abortion for a method failure (Table 4-2), many teens find these combined methods undesirable and, therefore, choose the pill. The pill is the next safest method (during the earlier years of a woman's life). It is also important to remember that the risk from the pill, provided that the patient is not at risk for other causes, is still significantly less than the risk of completing a pregnancy.

ORAL CONTRACEPTIVE PILLS

Most adolescents will choose the oral contraceptive for their method of birth control because of its low risk and failure rate, relief of cramps, and the ease of taking the pill without interfering with the spontaneity of in-

Table 4-2. Risk of Mortality/100,000 Nonsterile Women

	Age		
	15–19	20–24	40–44
No Control	35	37	141
Abortion	3	6	6
Pill/non-smoker	3	3	160
Pill/smoker	12	18	588
IUD	6	6	10
Condoms	6	8	2
Diaphragm	10	6	14
Condom and abortion	1	1	1
Rhythm	12	8	18

tercourse. Nevertheless, it is very important to individualize the needs of every adolescent, sick or well, when counseling for oral contraception. It is essential to do a complete history and physical examination, including weight, blood pressure monitoring, breast exam, and pelvic exam. The laboratory tests that are appropriate are a hemoglobin or hematocrit, urinalysis, Papanicolaou smear (yearly unless otherwise indicated), syphilis test (yearly), and culture for gonorrhea and chlamydia (at least every 6 months, perhaps alternately or whenever the clinical symptoms indicate). If there is a strong family history, cholesterol and triglycerides should be done. If everything is in favor of the pill, the patient should be instructed carefully in how to take the particular pill the physician is prescribing and how to deal with such things as breakthrough bleeding (reassurance); missing a pill (double up on the pills if one pill is missed; if two pills are missed, take all the missed pills but use a backup method of birth control); and nausea (take the pills with food and possibly at night before sleep).

The timing of follow-up visits depends on one's prediction of the compliance of the patient. It may be as often as monthly initially, at the discretion of the physician. The first follow-up visit for the compliant patient should be at 3 months for a weight and blood pressure check and discussion of any possible side effects of the pill. The subsequent visits, for a history and physical (including weight, blood pressure, breast exam, and pelvic exam), should be every 6 months.

Most of the current pills on the market are combination pills that contain both estrogen and progesterone. (There is a pill, called the "mini-pill," which contains only progesterone.) Table 4-3 contains a list of all the commonly available pills and their estrogen and progesterone content. The estrogen contained in the pills is either ethinyl estradiol or mestranol, which is metabolized in the liver to ethinyl estradiol; therefore, peak serum levels of ethinyl estradiol are lower after ingestion of mestranol than after one takes a pill containing ethinyl estradiol as its estrogen.[5] The 35-μg pills all

Table 4-3. Oral Contraceptives Available in the United States

Drug	Estrogen	(μg)	Progestin	(mg)
Combinations				
Demulen	ethinyl estradiol	50	ethynodiol diacetate	1
Ovral	ethinyl estradiol	50	norgestrel	0.5
Ovcon-50	ethinyl estradiol	50	norethindrone	1
Norinyl 1/50	mestranol	50	norethindrone	1
Ortho-Novum 1/50	mestranol	50	norethindrone	1
Demulen 1/35	ethinyl estradiol	35	ethynodiol diacetate	1
Norinyl 1/35	ethinyl estradiol	35	norethindrone	1
ON 1/35	ethinyl estradiol	35	norethindrone	1
Brevicon	ethinyl estradiol	35	northeindrone	0.5
Modicon	ethinyl estradiol	35	norethindrone	0.5
Ovcon-35	ethinyl estradiol	35	norethindrone	0.4
Lo-Ovral	ethinyl estradiol	30	norgestrel	0.3
Loestrin 1.5/30	ethinyl estradiol	30	norethindrone acetate	1.5
Nordette	ethinyl estradiol	30	levonorgestrel	0.15
Loestrin 1/20	ethinyl estradiol	20	norethindrone acetate	1
Ovrette			norgestrel	0.075
Nor-Q.D.			northeindrone	0.35
Micronor			norethindrone	0.35
ON 7/7/7	ethinyl estradiol	35	norethindrone	.5 × 7d .75× 7d 1.0 × 7d
TriNorinyl	ethinyl estradiol	35	norethindrone	.5 × 7d 1.0 × 7d .5 × 7d
Triphasil	ethinyl estradiol	30	levonorgestrel	.05 × 6d .075× 5d
TriLevlen		40		.125 ×10d

contain ethinyl estradiol, and the 50–100-μg pills contain either ethinyl estradiol or mestranol. Because some patients do not completely convert mestranol to ethinyl estradiol hepatically, it is difficult to compare the potency of these estrogens, which also can be affected by the progestins contained in the pills.

The combination pills suppress the ovarian–hypothalamic axis and, thus, inhibit ovulation, alter the endometrium to make implantation less likely, and make the cervical mucous more viscous.[6] The low-dose pills must be taken regularly and not missed, because they may be less suppressive to the hypothalamus.[7] The minipill, which contains only progesterone, is not felt to suppress the hypothalamus in exactly the same way, although in some patients the minipill blocks hypothalamic feedback, eliminating the luteinizing hormone (LH) surge. The minipill seems to work as a contraceptive—although not as effectively as the combination pill (the pregnancy rate is considerably higher: 1.5–3.0 pregnancies/100 woman-years)—by alteration

Table 4-4. Birth Control Pills

Minor side effects
  BTB, headaches, nausea, weight gain, mood change, acne, pill amenorrhea
Major side effects
  HBP, thromboembolism, strokes, cardiovascular disease, ↓ HDL-C
Possible benefits
  Less uterine and ovarian cancer, PID, less anemia, less cramps
Drug interactions
Cervical cancer

of the cervical mucous and the endometrium. The problem with the mini-pill is that some people bleed all the time and some are amenorrheic. Furthermore, there is no way to anticipate in advance who will fall into which category. Some patients are actually found to cycle on the minipill after a time.

In determining which pill to pick at first, most physicians now start with a 35-μg estrogen pill, and many will choose a triphasic progesterone pill, which approximates the endogenous hormones to stabilize the endometrium more effectively. The estrogen-dominant or progestin-dominant character of various pills must be considered when one is dealing with patients with specific problems, such as hirsutism, acne, oligomenorrhea, or with patients who suffer from specific estrogen symptoms, such as bloating or nausea. One must be very familiar with the side effects and contraindications of the pills before prescribing.

The side effects of the pill can be divided into major and minor ones, as shown in Table 4-4. Obviously, the major side effects, such as hepatic adenomas, hypertension, and other cardiovascular complications, are significant and require discontinuation of the pill. The pill is obviously not recommended for women with preexisting hypertension. It has been found that 1–5% of normotensive patients will develop elevated blood pressures (blood pressure>140/90) within weeks to several months of starting the pill.[8-11] This hormonally induced hypertension usually resolves within 2–12 weeks after discontinuation of the pill, during which time the patient should be encouraged to use another method of contraception. If the patient is unable to comply with this, for whatever reason, one could try using a significantly lower-dose pill such as Loestrin 1/20 or using the minipill and monitoring the patient's blood pressure frequently.

The patient who is at risk for any thromboembolic events on the basis of a previous history of such an event, eg, previous pulmonary embolism, or on the basis of a well-known medical problem, such as a hypercoaguable state, must not be considered a candidate for the birth control pill. For example, sickle cell anemia is a contraindication, although sickle cell trait is not. Significant varicosities are a contraindication, as is cyanotic heart disease. There has been an association of oral contraceptives and risk of stroke in several studies,[12–15] but these risks were increased further by other predisposing factors, such as cigarette smoking and hypertension. If a patient has a history of migraine headaches and refuses to use another method of contraception, then one would obviously discuss seriously with the patient the possibility that her headaches may get worse, and, if they do, she needs to contact the physician immediately. It goes without saying that this patient would do better with the very-low-dose pill or even the minipill. An absolute contraindication to the pill by most neurologists is ocular migraine. In such circumstances, an alternative method of birth control must be seriously considered.[16]

Since we know that the pills alter both carbohydrate and lipid metabolism, ideally one would want to encourage a person with diabetes mellitus to use an alternative method of birth control. Sometimes the reality is that it is a young teenager who will not use any other method. Because the risk to her life of carrying a pregnancy is great, she could be carefully monitored on a low-dose pill to see how she would do (one must carefully monitor insulin requirements although low-dose pills affect this less than higher-dose pills).[17] Lipid metabolism has been a current controversy with the birth control pills as it relates to the increasing incidence of cardiovascular complications. The estrogens seem not to be incriminated in this since they are felt to be protective and to increase high-density lipoprotein (HDL) cholesterol, but the progesterones do not escape scrutiny. Obviously, the risk is greater in older women who are smokers and perhaps have other risk factors, such as hypertension, family history of hyperlipoproteinemias, and/or a strong family history of cardiovascular disease or diabetes mellitus. We must be aware of the increased risk to adolescents who smoke, as well (Table 4-2). The studies done on both HDL and low-density lipoprotein (LDL) show that more potent progestins have been associated with increased LDL and decreased HDL cholesterols and, some might even say, an increased risk of coronary heart disease.[18,19] There continues to be much debate in the literature about this.

We are often faced with taking care of adolescents who, despite chronic medical problems or mental handicaps, are sexually active, as unlikely as that may seem to us. We must be very careful, in taking care of these patients, not to focus exclusively on the medical problems and ignore the broader picture. In counseling such a patient, we must first evaluate the potential of her becoming pregnant as best we can, then evaluate the risk of the birth control method in the presence of her disease, and, finally, consider the risk to her life of an unwanted pregnancy. If the patient is unable or unwilling to use a mechanical or chemical method, then we are faced with the risk of the low-dose pill. For example, the pill is felt to be contraindicated in patients with lupus erythematosus; however, we sometimes prescribe the low-dose pill for young adolescents with this disease who are reluctant to cooperate with another method and are at high risk for a pregnancy. The same rationale is true for a patient with epilepsy, but in this case the medications that she may be on for anticonvulsant therapy may increase the metabolism of the contraceptive steroids and place the patient at a greater risk of pill failure, especially if she should miss one pill.[20,21]

When one is prescribing the low-dose triphasic birth control pills, unless there is a specific problem, there probably is no real difficulty. There is no paucity of literature about varying progesterone concentrations and their effects. Many physicians support the use of one contraceptive over another. The important issue remains that one must talk to the patient and take a good personal as well as family history, examine the patient, and monitor the patient after prescribing any oral contraceptive. One must always be ready to reevaluate and change the prescription if necessary. The more commonly seen side effects, which are frequently minor but nevertheless very annoying to the patient, are the following: headaches, nausea, weight gain, breakthrough bleeding, acne, mood change, and pill amenorrhea. Frequently, these side effects can be dealt with in an anticipatory manner when one is prescribing the pill for the first time, since some of them are very predictable. Nausea and weight gain are estrogen symptoms and, therefore, can frequently be resolved by changing the estrogen content of the pill. For some people, breakthrough bleeding is the rule rather than the exception, especially in the first couple of months on the low-dose pill. If one warns the patient about the possible occurrence of this symptom and reassures the patient, it will frequently be a nonproblem. However, if breakthrough bleeding persists, then one may need to alter the estrogen or progesterone content. Earlier cycle bleeding may indicate an estrogen deficiency, and later cycle bleeding may indicate inadequate progesterone. Pill amenorrhea may indicate that the patient needs a higher-dose estrogen pill (only after the possibility of pregnancy is excluded). Because most women will feel more comfortable getting their periods every month than being anxious about a possible pregnancy, it is worthwhile to try to find a pill that allows the patient to have a withdrawal flow. One must explain clearly to the patient that her period may be much lighter than her normal flow off the pill and that she might even perceive it as spotting. For a patient with problem acne, it would not be prudent to prescribe a very androgenic pill, which might very well exacerbate an already annoying condition.

It is very important with teenagers to anticipate dissatisfaction with the pill, such as that produced by weight gain or breakthrough bleeding. Such anticipatory guidance may avert the patient's stopping the pill and suffering an unwanted pregnancy. In prescribing the pill, one may also talk about the noncontraceptive benefits of the pill, such as relief of dysmenorrhea, decreased flow during cycles, and decreased incidence of ovarian and endometrial cancer. Finally, it is important to realize that birth control pills can interfere with approximately 100 laboratory tests.[22] Some of the measurements that may not actually reflect the clinical state of the patient are the following: elevated sedimentation rate, elevated serum iron and total iron binding capacity, increased thyroxin (T4), decreased resin T3 (secondary to an increase in thyroid binding globulin), decreased haptoglobulin, and decreased serum folate, to name just a few of the more common tests affected.

INTRAUTERINE DEVICES

There are now only two intrauterine devices (IUDs) available in the United States. Progestasert (Alza) gradually releases progesterone.[23] Its particular difficulty is that it needs to be replaced yearly in addition to its having the other complications of the IUD. The newly released copper T 380A (ParaGard-GynoPharma) is the other available device.[24] The copper IUDs stimulate a mild inflammatory reaction in the uterus, decrease the viability of the sperm, and impair ovum transport. Many people cannot deal with the abnormal bleeding and cramping with the device, and there is some concern that this might be greater with the new copper T. The chief risk of the IUD is pelvic inflammatory disease (PID), which may lead to infertility. (Patients with multiple sex partners are at higher risk.) The other risks include perforation of the uterus on insertion, septic abortion if pregnancy occurs, and an increased incidence of ectopic pregnancies. The teenager, who is beginning her reproductive history, may have multiple sex partners and is certainly not a good candidate for this method of birth control, since it may make her infertile for the future and leave her with chronic pelvic pain from PID.

DIAPHRAGM

The use of female barriers obviously requires a motivated patient. This may not always be the case with the younger adolescent, who needs to be comfortable with her own body. The older, more mature adolescent in a committed relationship may be a much better candidate for the use of this method of contraception. When counseling the patient, one must talk about the possibility of dealing with an unwanted pregnancy and what options would be available.

The diaphragm is fitted by the health care provider, who must be patient. First, the adolescent patient must be given some sense of her own anatomy and how the diaphragm works. Then she must be fitted with the device and allowed to experience what it feels like when it is in place properly, covering her cervix. She must then be allowed to take it out and to insert it under supervision. The diaphragm should be checked again for positioning by the health care provider. The patient should be given both verbal and written instructions as to the use of the diaphragm, including the volume and timing of the use of the spermicidal jelly or cream. The teaching aids of the Ortho pelvic model and the Omni Health Communication cassettes are very helpful for the adolescent.

The patient is given the following instructions: 1) Although the diaphragm can be inserted up to 2 hours before intercourse, spermicidal cream or jelly must be inserted with each intercourse if more than 2 hours have elapsed. To do so, place 1 to 2 tsp of contraceptive jelly or cream in the cup of the diaphragm, and spread a small amount around the rim. 2) After insertion of the diaphragm, check to see if the cervix is covered by the device. 3) Leave the diaphragm in for at least 6 hours after the last intercourse (but ideally not more than 12 hours) and avoid douching after removing it. 4) After removal, wash the diaphragm with mild soap and dry completely. (Dust with corn starch, if desired.) 5) Before each use, check the diaphragm for holes by holding it up to the light, and check around the spring to make sure there are no cracks. 6) Replace the device at least every 2 years or as soon as there is any evidence of a crack and thinning of the rubber. 7) Have the diaphragm checked following extreme weight changes and at the annual gynecologic visit.

CERVICAL CAP

The cervical cap is similar to the diaphragm, except that it is smaller and consists of a rigid plastic cup that holds the spermicidal agent. It is applied directly on the cervix and is held in place by suction. Its failure rates are not dissimilar to those of the diaphragm and, in some practices, are felt to be higher. The cap has recently been approved by the Food and Drug Administration (FDA) and will be available more widely now. But its limitations remain: It takes a long time to fit a cervical cap and counsel a patient in its proper use. Although the cap can be left in place for an extended period of time, which varies depending on the type of cap, not everyone can use the cap. Furthermore, there is some concern about changes in the Papanicolaou smear in cap users. The younger adolescent does not seem to be a very good candidate for this method of contraception.

CONDOM AND CHEMICAL METHOD

The advantage of the condoms and spermicidal contraceptive agents is that they are easily available over the counter. In addition, we no longer talk about oral contraceptives without also talking about the use of the condoms; the former is for birth control, and the latter is for life (AIDS) control. It is important to instruct the male about the proper use of the condom and to encourage the use of latex condoms. Although there are many types and brands of spermicidal agents available, the active ingredient in all of these is nonoxynol 9. Nevertheless, it is probably a good idea to mention some specific types and brand names: foams (Emko, Delfen), suppositories (Encare

Oval, Semicid, Intercept), individual applications (Vaginal Contraceptive Foam—VCF, Conceptrol).

SPONGE

The Today sponge is a small, round sponge impregnated with nonoxynol 9. It can be bought over the counter and can be used for 24 hours. Like the spermicides, it must also be used in conjunction with the condom to make it a more effective form of contraception and to protect against AIDS.

THE "MORNING AFTER" PILL

This is certainly not a recommended routine method of birth control but is to be used in the event of a personal or technical failure of another method of contraception. The preferred pill in many rape protocols is Ovral, which is taken in the dosage of two tablets stat. within 48 hours, then two tablets 12 hours later.[25,26]

FUTURE DEVELOPMENTS IN CONTRACEPTION

Because of the lack of a perfect (foolproof, without limitation and side effects) method of birth control, researchers are constantly looking to improve methods of contraception. Injectable progestins (Depo Provera and Norethindrone enanthate) are not approved by the FDA. Subcutaneous hormonal implants (Norplant), which have been reported to be effective for 5 years of contraception, are not available for use in the United States. Because of the occurrence of irregular bleeding, this method is not very attractive to most women. Vaccines, LH/RH analogs, and the long-awaited male contraception are still coming attractions in contraceptive technology.

REFERENCES

1. Zelnick, Kantner: Fam Plann Perspect 1980;12:230.
2. Emans SJ, Goldstein DP: Birth control. Pediatr Adolesc Gynecol 1982.
3. Emans SJ, Grace E, et al: Adolescents' compliance with the use of oral contraceptives. JAMA 1987;257:3377.
4. Zabin LS, Hirsch MB, et al: Evaluation of a pregnancy program for urban teenagers. Fam Plann Perspect 1986;18:119.
5. Brenner PF, Goebelsmann U, et al: Serum levels of ethinyl estradiol following its ingestion alone or in oral contraceptive formulations. Contraception 1980;22:85.
6. Garcia GR: The oral contraceptive: An appraisal and review. Am J Med Sci 1967;253:718.
7. Scott JZ, Kletsky OA, Brenner PF, et al: Comparison of the effects of contraceptive steroid formations containing two doses of estrogen on pituitary function. Fertil Steril 1978;30:141.
8. Greenblatt D, Kochweser J: Oral contraceptives and hypertension. Obstet Gynecol 1974;44:412.
9. Russell RP, Sullivan MA: The pill and hypertension. Johns Hopkins Med J 1970;127:287.

10. Crane MG, Harris JJ, Winsor W: Hypertension: Oral contraceptive agents and conjugated estrogens. Ann Intern Med 1971;74:13.
11. Weinberger AM: Oral contraceptives and hypertension. Hosp Pract 1975;10:65.
12. Inman W, Vessey MP, Westerholm B, et al: Thromboembolic disease and the steroidal content of oral contraceptive pills: A report to the committee on safety of drugs. Br Med J 1970;2:203.
13. Boston Collaborative Drug Surveillance Program. Oral contraceptives and venous thromboembolic disease: Surgically confirmed gallbladder disease and breast tumors. Lancet 1973;i:1399.
14. Collaborative Group in the study of stroke in young women. Oral contraception and increased risk of cerebral ischemia or thrombosis. N Engl J Med 1973;288:871.
15. Sartwell PE, Masi AT, Arthes FG, et al: Thromboembolism and oral contraceptives: An epidemiologic case-control study. Am J Epidemiol 1969;90:365.
16. Nicolson DH, Walsh FB: Oral contraceptives and neuro-ophthalmic disorders. J Reprod Med 1969;3:37.
17. Spellacy WN, Buhi WC, Birk SA: Carbohydrate metabolism with three months of low-estrogen contraceptive use. Am J Obstet Gynecol 1980;138:151.
18. Wallace RB, Tamir I, Heiss G, et al: Plasma lipids, lipoproteins, and blood pressure in female adolescents using oral contraceptives. J Pediatr 1979;95:1055.
19. Bradley DD, Wingerd J, Petitti DB, et al: Serum high-density-lipoprotein cholesterol in women using oral contraceptives, estrogens, and progestins. N Engl J Med 1978;299:17.
20. Janz D, Schmidt D: Anti-epileptic drugs and failure of oral contraceptives. Lancet 1974;i:1113.
21. Laengner H, Detering K: Anti-epileptic drugs and failure of oral contraceptives. Lancet 1974;ii:600.
22. Miale JB, Kent JW: The effects of oral contraceptives on the results of laboratory tests. Am J Obstet Gynecol 1974;120:264.
23. Progestasert—a new intrauterine contraceptive device. Med Lett Drugs Ther 1976;18:65.
24. New copper IUD. Med Lett Drugs Ther 1988;30:760.
25. Dixon GW, Schlesselman JJ, Ory HW, et al: Ethinyl estradiol and conjugated estrogens as post coital contraceptives. JAMA 1980;244:1336.
26. Morris JM, Van Wagenen G: Interception: The use of postovulatory estrogens to prevent implantation. Am J Obstet Gynecol 1973;115:101.

The Insulin-dependent Diabetic Adolescent: A Contraceptive Dilemma

Jacques Robert Mailloux, MD, FRCP, and
Donald Peter Goldstein, MD

The modern teenager enjoys an active sexual life, and adolescents with insulin-dependent diabetes mellitus (IDDM) are no exception. The most recent national survey of metropolitan youth revealed that the mean age of first intercourse for females is 16.2 years and that 16% of them will have experienced a pregnancy before they reach adulthood.[1] In fact, this country's actual teenage pregnancy rate of 1 million per year is the highest in any developed country in the world! Our society has obviously failed to deal adequately with issues of sexuality and continues to ignore these overpowering statistics.

Diabetes mellitus affects some 100,000 individuals under age 20 in the United States and is one of the most common endocrine disorders of youth.[2] The fact that diabetic adolescents are more closely followed than most other teenagers for medical reasons should provide us with a unique opportunity to discuss openly and inquire actively about sexuality and contraception. Regrettably, these topics are often ignored when care is being provided for the chronically ill adolescent, and they receive much less attention than they actually deserve in the current context of preventive medicine.

Counseling implies education, not judgment. We preach and judge abundantly but too often leave out teaching and understanding. Young teenagers do not equate coitus with eventual pregnancy. Misinformation about contraception being wrong or dangerous is perpetuated. In fact, there is no evidence that increased sexual knowledge changes the likelihood that teenagers will have sexual intercourse. However, there is evidence that knowledge about contraception leads to increased usage and a decrease in the teenage pregnancy rate.[3] Ideally, contraception counseling should start

Presented in part at the Annual Meeting of the American Diabetes Association held in Anaheim, California, on June 21, 1986.

Clinical Practice of Gynecology: **3**, 52–60, 1989

ISSN 1043-3198/89/$3.50
655 Avenue of the Americas, New York, NY 10010

early and involve the school, the church, and the family. The physician should encourage and be willing to assist the adolescent in obtaining parental permission. Acceptance of and adherence to a contraceptive plan by an adolescent is more likely to occur in a supportive family situation.[4] On the other hand, although parent involvement is encouraged, the courts have ruled that family planning services for teenagers may remain confidential, and this point should be stressed in dealing with adolescents. Confidentiality, accessibility, and nonjudgmental approach form the basis for a trusting patient–physician relationship. The percentage of effective contraceptive use at first intercourse is mainly age dependent: 31% for 15-year-old teenagers compared to 62% at 18 years of age.[5] Therefore, it must become routine for the health care provider to inquire about sexual activity as part of the routine history in order to increase the likelihood that the adolescent will use contraception at first intercourse.

Compliance is another important factor that has to be considered in providing contraception for adolescents. Even if we assume that IDDM patients are more likely to be compliant to a prescribed regimen, we have to remember that contraceptive use by teenagers is influenced by age, frequency of intercourse, autonomy of the patient in making and paying for a clinic appointment, and acceptance of the method picked at the first clinic visit.[6]

Finally, we have to remember that some teenagers may lack the maturity or financial resources to use contraception regularly and to keep follow-up appointments. In fact, side effects of any contraceptive method in adolescent patients typically lead to discontinuance rather than a clinic visit or a phone call.[7]

The purpose of this chapter is to review the current status of the main contraceptive methods available to the IDDM adolescent and to discuss the pros and cons of each modality. Counseling by a friendly, concerned, health care provider will allow each patient to make her own choice based on a sound understanding of the mechanisms, benefits, and risks of each method.

HORMONAL CONTRACEPTION

Combined Oral Contraceptive Steroids (COCS)

The birth control pill (BCP) is currently one of the most frequently used reversible methods of fertility control in the teenage population. This is due in large part to its low overall failure rate of 2% in typical users.[8] The failure rate is age related, since in typical users under age 22, the figure rises to 4.7%.[9]

In recent years, there has been a decline in the use of birth control pills because of overemphasis on their side effects and adverse publicity in the lay press. In fact, the mortality rate from pregnancy and childbirth in the 15–19-year age group of 12.9 deaths per 100,000 live births far exceeds the 0.3 and 2.2 deaths per 100,000 users of BCP per year for nonsmokers and smokers, respectively.[10] We believe that the noncontraceptive benefits of the pill should also be emphasized. It is well known that BCP reduces the incidence of irregular or excessive periods, dysmenorrhea, functional ovarian cysts, salpingitis, ectopic pregnancy, benign breast disease, anemia, and endometrial and ovarian cancer.[11–14]

Most clinicians are justifiably concerned about the potentially adverse effects of even slight alterations of lipid and carbohydrate metabolism induced by BCP on the diabetic adolescent. Data from the Bogalusa Heart Study shows that metabolic risk factors, such as high low-density lipoprotein (LDL) cholesterol serum levels, are correlated with atherosclerosis very early in life.[15] Therefore, youth does not appear to offer protection from initiation of cardiovascular pathology, and, consequently, uncomplicated IDDM is considered a strong relative contraindication to BCP use, while complicated IDDM stands as an absolute contraindication. In the last 10 years, the growing concern about long-term side effects of BCP, especially with regard to alterations in carbohydrate and lipid metabolism, has triggered the development of newer combined BCP with lower steroid content, high efficacy, and minimal metabolic changes. There are a number of BCP currently on the market containing 30–35 μg of ethinyl estradiol (EE), a level regarded as the lowest that can reliably prevent pregnancy.[16] The only formulation with 20 μg of EE (Lo-Estrin 1/20) has been shown to have reduced contraceptive effectiveness as well as a high incidence of irregular bleeding.[16,17] However, there are other differences in these newer "sub-50" pills, and they lie in their different progestin content.

Effects on Carbohydrate Metabolism

The effect of the pill on carbohydrate metabolism was originally thought to be related to high levels of estrogen (80–100 μg). Since the appearance of the newer "sub-50" formulation, Spellacy and colleagues[18–20] have shown in various clinical studies that estrogen has no significant effect on carbohydrate metabolism, but the type and dosage of the progestogen used plays an important and previously underestimated role. In fact, norgestrel-containing "sub-50" formulations (Lo-Ovral, Nordette) have repeatedly been found to alter carbohydrate metabolism to a greater degree than those containing norethindrone (Ovcon-35, Brevicon, Modicon, Norinyl 1/35, Ortho-Novum 1/35).[21,22] Even the newest multiphasic formulations containing levonorgestrel (Triphasil, Trilevlen) were found to cause an increase in both the plasma glucose and insulin levels while formulations containing varying amounts of norethindrone (ON 777, Tri-Norinyl) caused no significant changes.[23–25] From this data, it appears that low doses of a low-activity progestin, such as norethindrone, does not have a significant impact on carbohydrate metabolism.

Effects on Lipid Metabolism

With the advent of the newest "low-dose" combination BCP, the concept of a lipid-neutral pill has recently evolved. Because estrogen and progestin have counteracting effects on HDL-cholesterol levels, early studies on lipid metabolism were confusing and often not designed to consider confounding factors like cigarette smoking.

Estrogen and progestin affect lipoprotein levels differently. Low-dose estrogen increases HDL-cholesterol and decreases LDL-cholesterol levels, thus providing a protective effect against atherosclerosis. On the other hand, androgenic progestin decreases high-density lipoprotein (HDL) cholesterol and increases LDL cholesterol, which would tend to promote heart disease. Thus, the impact on various lipoprotein levels is determined by the estrogen–progestin potency ratio in a given pill as well as by the androgenicity of the progestin used.[26] Wahl and colleagues[27] found the lowest levels of HDL cholesterol and the highest levels of LDL cholesterol with norgestrel (Lo-Ovral, Trilevlen, Triphasil) and norethindrone acetate (Lo-Estrin)-containing products.[27] Norethindrone-containing formulations, on the other hand, did not have a negative effect on either HDL or LDL cholesterol levels.[24,27] Recent research has shown that progestin can also modify the composition of the total HDL cholesterol by altering the relative amount of HDL_2 and HDL_3 subfractions.[25] It is the HDL_2 fraction that provides the beneficial effect against heart disease, whereas HDL_3 has no protective role.[28] The birth control pill may then affect a patient's lipid profile even though the total HDL cholesterol remains unchanged. For example, while one study determined that norgestrel-containing Triphasil did not affect total HDL levels,[29] another study found that this combination led to a decrease in HDL_2 and an increase in HDL_3 cholesterol that increases heart risks.[30] In contrast, various norethindrone-containing BCP did not appear to alter levels of HDL_2 cholesterol, further supporting the use of this progestin to lessen the metabolic impact.[31,32] Kraus,[32] in a small randomized study, showed that both total HDL_3 and HDL_2 subfractions were increased in women treated with 35 µg of EE in combination with 0.4 mg of norethindrone (Ovcon 35).

Of the currently used progestin in low-dose formulations, it has been shown conclusively that norethindrone had the smallest impact on both carbohydrate and lipid metabolism. Therefore, it is our recommendation that IDDM teenagers with uncomplicated disease, who require highly effective contraception, be put on low-dose norethindrone-containing BCP. Our first choice would be Ovcon 35, which provides 8.4 mg of norethindrone per cycle, followed by Brevicon or Modicon with 10.0 mg/cycle,

TriNorinyl with 15 mg/cycle, and, last, Ortho Novum 777 with 15.75 mg/ cycle.

Regular medical examinations at 6-month intervals is mandatory for IDDM women on the pill in order to identify early retinopathy, nephropathy, or a cardiovascular complication that would absolutely contraindicate further usage.[33] It would also seem reasonable to restrict its use to patients without additional risk factors like smoking, hypertension, or a family history of vascular disease.[33] The very prolonged use of BCP (>5 years) should be discouraged in diabetic patients, and the importance of early pregnancy with prepregnancy counseling and early sterilization should be stressed. Finally, serial determinations of lipoprotein levels should be considered for additional safety.

The Minipill or Progestin-only Pill

The minipill contains the same synthetic progestins that are used in the combined oral contraceptive but in smaller doses and without any estrogens. Two formulations are marketed in the United States, one containing 0.35 mg of norethindrone (Micronor, Nor-Q-D) and the other, 0.075 mg of dl-norgestrel (Ovrette). The progestogen dose is lower than in any combined oral contraceptives currently available. Since progestin-induced metabolic side effects are dose-related and mainly seen with norgestrel, it is expected that norethindrone-containing pills be of special interest to IDDM women.

The progestin-only pill acts at three different levels: rendering the cervical mucus thick, impairing the normal development of the endometrium, and interfering with the corpus luteum. While they are on these pills, approximately 40% of women show a normal ovulatory pattern, and 20% shift back and forth from ovulatory to anovulatory cycles, and 20% are consistently anovulatory.[34]

The first-year failure rate of typical users on the minipill is 2.5%, which falls between the combination oral contraceptive and the IUD. Ovrette may be associated with a slightly lower failure rate, given its higher relative potency. Pregnancy rates are highest in the first 6 months on the minipill, and a back-up barrier method is indicated during this time. Pregnancy rates are the lowest when progestin-only pills are substituted for combination oral contraceptives.

There is actually no evidence that the minipill disrupts carbohydrate metabolism, and for that reason it would appear to be ideal for use in IDDM women.[34] Insulin requirements, blood pressure, coronary and cerebrovascular disease, retinopathy, and clotting factors have not been affected by the taking of these preparations. Of particular importance for diabetics, the minipill has little or no effect on lipid metabolism, including HDL levels.[34] Probably the main disadvantage, which limits the more widespread use of the progestin-only pill, is the irregular bleeding pattern seen in about 20–

30% of users. Abnormal bleeding patterns usually improve spontaneously with time, and more severe cases are often controlled by either doubling the dose for 1 month or by using a short course of estrogen by mouth (Premarin 2.5 mg one per day for 1 week).

The minipill should be started on day one of the cycle and taken every day, ideally at the same time. Irregular cycles are the most common reason for discontinuation, so patients should be adequately counseled beforehand to improve compliance. A moderate gain in weight of 3–6 lb is also frequently seen at the beginning of therapy because of water retention, and teenagers are occasionally very distressed by this side effect. Finally, if a period of amenorrhea lasts more than 45 days, a pregnancy test should be promptly ordered.

INTRAUTERINE CONTRACEPTIVE DEVICE (IUCD)

The IUCD is mentioned here only to condemn its use in any teenager, particularly if diabetic. Women using IUCDs are at an increased risk of developing pelvic inflammatory disease, infertility, and ectopic pregnancy. Because of these factors, IUCD use should be actively discouraged in women who have not had any children[36] and who are more likely to be exposed to sexually transmitted diseases (STDs). Furthermore, recent reports suggest that IDDM patients using IUCDs have an unexpected high failure rate.[37] The reported first-year failure rate in typical users is 5%.

Although an interesting concept, the progestin-releasing IUCD (Progestasert), with its large diameter and need for yearly replacement, is hardly fit for widespread use in adolescents. Also, a higher ectopic pregnancy rate reported for the Progestasert is of concern.

Some may consider the IUCD appealing for the noncompliant adolescent or when oral contraceptives are contraindicated. The advantages of the IUCD (ie, compliance and lack of metabolic side effects) have to be weighed against impairment of future fertility.[38]

BARRIER METHODS

Barrier methods certainly offer to the IDDM patient two main advantages: They are devoid of any systemic or metabolic side effects, and they afford some protection against STDs so prevalent in this age group.

On the other hand, unacceptably high failure rates have been observed in typical youth users mainly because of misuse or failure to use the method at all. The pregnancy rates are so variable and dependent upon patient compliance and motivation that comparison is worthless.

Generally, these methods require excellent communication between partners and some degree of anticipation of coitus. The condom, eg, needs an understanding partner and does require skillful and constant use to be effective. With older or very well-motivated adolescents, successful diaphragm use has been documented by Lowe and associates.[39]

Spermicidal suppositories, foam, or sponges are available over-the-counter. These techniques are popular with adolescents who engage in intercourse infrequently; however, it is our opinion that only exceptional teenagers can reliably use barrier methods for contraception.

CONCLUSION

In summary, the best contraceptive method for an individual diabetic teenager is the one with which she feels most comfortable and will consequently use adequately. Contraception in IDDM patients must strike a balance between benefits and risks. Above all, it should be remembered that the methods discussed above are far safer for teenagers than an unplanned pregnancy and childbirth! Concerns regarding the long-term metabolic side effects of the pill have been voiced, and for now the low-dose, norethindrone-containing BCP or the progestin-only pill seems to overcome most objections. In the near future, a slow-releasing ultra-low-dose progestin device (subdermal implants or vaginal ring) will probably become the elusive ideal method as far as the metabolic impact is concerned for the IDDM patient. In the meantime, we must continue to provide teenagers with a confidential nonjudgmental approach that will permit them to make their own informed choice regarding available methods.

REFERENCES

1. Zelnik M, Kantner JF: Sexual activity, contraception use and pregnancy among metropolitan-area teenagers: 1971–1979. Fam Plann Perspect 1980;12:230–237.
2. Neinstein LS, Katz B: Contraceptive use in the chronically ill adolescent female: Part I. J Adolesc Health Care 1986;7:123–133.
3. Committee on Adolescence: Sexuality, contraception, and the media. Pediatrics 1986;78:535–536.
4. ACOG Technical Bulletin: The adolescent obstetric-gynecologic patient. Number 94, July, 1986.
5. Kulig JW: Adolescent contraception: An update. Pediatrics 1985;77:675–680.
6. Litt IF, Cuskey WR, Rudd S: Identifying adolescents at risk for noncompliance with contraceptive therapy. J Pediatr 1980;96:742–745.
7. Baldwin W: Adolescent pregnancy and childbearing: Rates, trends and research findings from the Center for Population Research, National Institute for Child Health and Human Development. Bethesda, MD, NICHD, 1986.
8. Shirm A, Trussel TJ, Menken J, Grady W: Contraceptive failure in the United States: The impact of racial, economic and demographic factors. Fam Plann Perspect 1982;14:68–75.
9. Ory HW, Forrest JD, Lincoln R: Making choices: Evaluating the health risks and benefits of birth control methods. New York: The Alan Guttmacher Institute, 1983.
10. Ory HW: Mortality associated with fertility and fertility control: 1983. Fam Plann Perspect 1983;15:57–63.
11. Mishell DR: Noncontraceptive health benefits of oral steroidal contraceptives. Am J Obstet Gynecol 1982;142:804–816.

12. Ory HW: The noncontraceptive health benefits from oral contraceptive use. Fam Plann Perspect 1982;14:182–184.

13. Division of Reproductive Health, Center for Health Promotion and Education, Center for Disease Control, DHHS: Oral contraceptive use and the risk of endometrial cancer. JAMA 1983;249:1600–1604.

14. Oral contraceptive use and the risk of ovarian cancer. JAMA 1983;249:1596–1599.

15. Newman WP III, Freedman DS, Voors AW, et al: Relation of serum lipoprotein levels and systolic blood pressure to early atherosclerosis: The Bogalusa Heart Study. N Engl J Med 1986;314:138.

16. Hatcher RA, et al: Contraceptive technology 1986–1987, 13th rev ed. Irvington Publishers, Inc.

17. Speroff L: The formulation of oral contraceptives: Does the amount of estrogen make any clinical difference? Johns Hopkins Med J 1982;150:170.

18. Spellacy WN, Buhi WC, Birk SA: Prospective studies of carbohydrate metabolism in "normal" women using norgestrel for eighteen months. Fertil Steril 1981;35:167.

19. Spellacy WN, Facog WC, Buhi MS, et al: Effects of norethindrone on carbohydrate and lipid metabolism. Obstet Gynecol 1975;46:560.

20. Spellacy WN, Buhi WC, Birk SA: Carbohydrate metabolism prospectively studied in women using a low-estrogen oral contraceptive for six months. Contraception 1979;20:137.

21. Wynn V: Effect of duration of low dose oral contraceptive administration on carbohydrate metabolism. Am J Obstet Gynecol 1982;142:739.

22. Wynn V, Godsland I: Effects of oral contraceptives on carbohydrate metabolism. J Reprod Med 1986;31(suppl):892.

23. Vermeulen A, Thiery M: Metabolic effects of the multiphasic oral contraceptive Trigynon. Contraception 1982;26:505.

24. Rabe T, Runnebaum B, Hageloch W, et al: Influence of a norethindrone containing multiphasic pill on carbohydrate and lipid metabolism. Contracept Delivery Syst 1984;5:50.

25. Ellis JS: Multiphasic oral contraceptives, efficacy and metabolic impact. J Reprod Med 1987;32:1,28.

26. Tikkanen MJ, Nikkila EA: Oral contraceptive and lipoprotein metabolism. J Reprod Med 1986;31(suppl):898.

27. Wahl P, Walden C, Knopp R, et al: Effect of estrogen/progestin potency on lipid/lipoprotein cholesterol. N Engl J Med 1983;308:862.

28. Miller NE, Hammett F, Saltissi S, et al: Relation of angiographically defined coronary artery disease to plasma lipoprotein subfraction and apolipoprotein. Br Med J 1981;282:1741.

29. Briggs MH: Implication and assessment of metabolic effects of oral contraceptives. New considerations in oral contraception. New York: BMI Publications, 1982.

30. Marz W, et al: Effect of oral contraceptives on serum lipoprotein patterns in healthy women. Advances in fertility control and treatment of sterility. Proc Sympos 11th World Congress, Dublin, 1984.

31. Stubblefield PG: Selection of steroid combinations for oral contraceptives of maximum benefit. J Reprod Med 1986;31(suppl):922.

32. Krauss RM, Roy S, Mishell DR, et al: Effects of two low dose oral contraceptives on serum lipids and lipoprotein subclasses. J Obstet Gynecol 1983;145:446.

33. Steel JM: Prepregnancy counseling and contraception in the insulin-dependent diabetic patient. Clin Obstet Gynecol 1985;28:553–566.

34. Graham S, Fraser IS: The progestogen-only mini-pill. Contraception 1982;26:373–388.

35. Shirm A, Trunell TJ, Manken J, Grady W: Contraceptive failure in the United States: The impact of social, economic and demographic factors. Fam Plann Perspect 1982;14:68–75.

36. Speroff L: Contraception for adolescents. Postgrad Obstet Gynecol 1983;3:14.

37. Gosden C, Ross A, Steel J, et al: Intrauterine contraceptive devices in diabetic women. Lancet 1982;530–535.

38. Kulig JW, Rauh JL, Burket RL, et al: Experience with the copper 7 intrauterine device in an adolescent population. J Pediatr 1980;96:746–750.
39. Lane ME, et al: Successful use of the diaphragm and jelly by a young population: Report of a clinical study. Fam Plann Perspect 1976;8:81–86.

CHAPTER 6

An Approach to Adolescent Pregnancy

Paul von Oeyen, MD, and Laurence E. Lundy, MD

Adolescent pregnancy continues to be a major health concern in the United States, with over 500,000 births each year to mothers under 20 years of age.[1] Compared to the great majority of other developed countries, teenage fertility (birth rates, abortion rates, and total pregnancy rates) is considerably higher in the United States.[2] As shown in Figure 6-1, the differences in teenage birth rates between the United States and five other developed countries are most striking in the youngest age groups.

The increased risk of poor pregnancy outcome and greater frequency of low birth weight and infant mortality has been repeatedly demonstrated for the adolescent gravida.[3–11] There are many potentially confounding factors, however, which may be more significant than age per se. These include socioeconomic status, race, nutrition, education, and utilization and availability of health care. This chapter will consider several risk factors associated with adolescent pregnancy and discuss methods for dealing with adolescent pregnancy that may improve obstetric and neonatal outcome.

Although the increase in numbers of births to adolescents in the 1960s and early 1970s has been viewed with alarm as an epidemic of teenage pregnancy, the actual birth rates during this time were declining (91.0 births per 1000 women age 15–19 in 1960 to 69.7 in 1970).[12] These seemingly contradictory statistics are the result of the post-World War II baby boom, which produced a peak teenage population in the late 1960s and early 1970. This increased number of teenagers resulted in more adolescent births in spite of a falling birth rate. The annual total of adolescent births is now declining, and the birth rate has continued to decline (52.5 per 1000 women age 15–19 in 1978).[12] The fall in the number of adolescent births has been primarily concentrated in the older age groups (Table 6-1).[1,12] Unfortu-

Clinical Practice of Gynecology: **3,** 61–71, 1989
© 1989 Elsevier Science Publishing Co., Inc.
655 Avenue of the Americas, New York, NY 10010

ISSN 1043-3198/89/$3.50

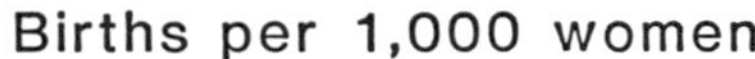
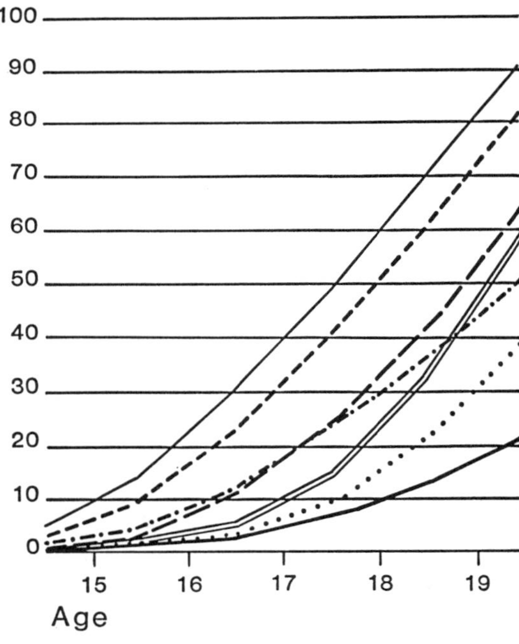

FIGURE 6-1 ____________
Births per 1,000 women under age 20, selected countries, 1981. Adapted with permission from Jones et al: Teen-aged pregnancy in developed countries: Determinant and policy implications. Fam Plann Perspect 1985; 17:53.

nately, it is the younger adolescents, aged 15 or less, that have the greatest risk in their first pregnancies, and are also most likely to have multiple births before the age of 20.

BIOMEDICAL RISKS

The issue of the requirement of biologic maturity for optimal pregnancy outcome has been controversial. If there are certain biologic factors, such as small pelvic size in young adolescent age groups, that are fixed in their influence on pregnancy outcome, there will be a limit to the possibility of limiting excess risk in adolescent pregnancy.

Table 6-1. Births per 1,000 Women 14–19 Years of Age: United States 1960–1981

Period	Age					
	14	15	16	17	18	19
1960–64	5.4	17.8	40.2	75.8	122.7	169.2
1970	6.6	19.2	38.8	66.6	98.3	126.0
1978	6.3	17.2	32.7	52.4	72.2	88.0
1981	5.4	14.1	30.4	49.8	71.0	92.1

From: 1960–1978: Baldwin; Adolescent pregnancy and childbearing—an overview. 1981;5:1. 1981: National Center for Health Statistics: Advance Report of Final Natality Statistics, 1981. Vital Health 1983; 32,9 (suppl).

The concept of gynecologic age attempts to relate the problems of adolescent pregnancy, at least in the youngest ages, to gynecologic maturity. Gynecologic age is the difference between the mother's age at delivery and her age at menarche.

In two studies, a gynecologic age of 2 years or less was associated with higher rates of low birth weight babies (<2,500 g).[13,14] Unfortunately, the use of the concept of gynecologic age may not be reliable, since many patients are uncertain about the precise age of menarche.[15]

Moerman[16] related low gynecologic age in young adolescents to small pelvic size when compared to a normal 18-year-old control group. The pelvic basin appears to grow slowly but continuously throughout late adolescence. Long bone growth, on the other hand, rapidly decelerates in the first year after menarche. Thus, one might expect a higher frequency of cephalopelvic disproportion in young gravid adolescents. In several studies examining this, however, only one indicated a higher cesarean section rate.[6,7,17–20]

Anemia, urinary tract infection, abruptio placentae, pregnancy-induced hypertension, and even maternal mortality have all been described in greater frequency in teenage pregnancy.[7,21–23] Menkin,[21] however, has shown that an apparent increase in teenage mortality was seen only in nonwhite adolescents and appears to be more related to race than to age. Most of the other risks are more clearly related to nutritional, social, and medical care access factors than to adolescent age.

Pregnancy-induced hypertension (preeclampsia) may be found in 15–40% of teenage pregnancies and is the most prevalent medical complication.[23] Although many studies have described high rates of preeclampsia in black adolescents,[3,7,10] pregnancy-induced hypertension is prevalent in all low-socioeconomic teenage groups. Early diagnosis and treatment of preeclampsia in teenagers may be delayed because their baseline blood pressures are generally lower, and a significant rise may occur without reaching the traditional "abnormal" level of 140/90 mmHg. Emphasis should be placed on the importance of suspecting pregnancy-induced hypertension when there have been increases in systolic or diastolic pressures of 30 mmHg and 15 mmHg, respectively, regardless of these having reached 140/90 mmHg.[24] Teenagers are at higher risk for pregnancy-induced hypertension likely on the basis of their being primigravidas and possibly on the immunologic basis of first exposure to antigens of paternal origin.[25]

MULTIPARITY

Many studies of adolescent pregnancy have lumped together all teenagers and have not separated out the very young or those with repeat pregnancies. McCormick and associates[26] identified two groups of adolescent mothers as being at an especially high risk for poor pregnancy outcome: young nulliparous teenagers 16 years of age or less, and 18–19-year-old multiparas. The high neonatal mortality rates in these groups were due mainly to higher proportions of low-birth-weight infants. Jekel and associates[8] also reported a high frequency of prematurity and perinatal mortality in teenage mothers experiencing second and third pregnancies. These reports concerning the multipara are in contrast to those in the general population, where second-born infants are less likely to be at low birth weight. Clearly, the parous teenager is at special high risk and requires careful intervention for family planning, nutrition, and general health services. The special prenatal programs often provided for teenagers in a first pregnancy should be made available for subsequent pregnancies as well.

SOCIOECONOMIC AND RACIAL FACTORS

Studies that have been controlled for social and economic background have shown very little increased risk for the pregnant adolescent.[9,28–30] Miller and Merritt,[31] studying a white population, showed no difference in the rate of low-birth-weight infant births to teenagers compared to mothers 20 years and older, after excluding "behavioral" conditions and medical complicating factors. The "behavioral" conditions listed included low prepregnancy weight for height, low maternal weight gain in pregnancy, lack of prenatal care, cigarette smoking, and use of addicting drugs or large amounts of alcohol during pregnancy. The medical complications included preeclampsia or other hypertension, severe vaginal bleeding, chronic disease or severe anemia (hemoglobin<10 g/dL), and polyhydramnios or oligohydramnios.[32] These studies suggest that the "behavioral" conditions and medical complications were more powerful predictors of infant birth weight less than the age of the mother alone.

Elster,[33] using multivariate analysis, showed that the risk for primiparous women having a small-for-gestational-age infant was more strongly related to late prenatal care than to young maternal age (12–14 years). Young teenagers who began prenatal care in the first trimester had rates of small-for-gestational-age infants (5%) similar to those of older teenagers and adults (6%) who also began care early. In the same study, young multiparous teenagers, regardless of when prenatal care began, were at increased risk for having a small-for-gestational-age infant when compared to adults. Both prenatal care and parity appear to have important influences on pregnancy outcome in adolescents.

Race has been found to be an important factor in pregnancy outcome. Many studies of adolescent pregnancy risks, however, have had disproportionately large numbers of black teenagers.[10,32,34,35] Infants of black adolescent mothers have been reported to be at higher risk for both neonatal and late infant deaths.[36,37] Although it has been generally assumed that the relationship of race to socioeconomic status is the main contributor to risk,[38] recent infant mortality data have suggested higher risks for blacks even after socioeconomic and educational differences were corrected for.[39]

Young women of lower socioeconomic status are more likely to be chronically undernourished, with poor nutritional and personal hygiene practices during pregnancy. They may have more gynecologic and urinary tract infections, smoke and drink more, and, in general, comply poorly with prenatal health care. Since the young adolescent who becomes pregnant and bears her child is likely to be "poor, black, unmarried, and not receive adequate prenatal care",[38] it is not surprising that there are greater risks for poor perinatal outcome.

PSYCHOSOCIAL RISKS

The young adolescent is facing the challenges and conflicts of her own psychosocial development. The additional stresses of pregnancy and parenting are frequently disruptive of this maturation process. Numerous studies have shown that adolescent parents and particularly the multipara are more likely to drop out of school and complete less formal education than teenagers who postpone parenthood, even when groups are matched for race, socioeconomic status, and academic aptitude.[40,41] On the other hand, a return to school after childbirth has been shown to be the best indicator of whether an adolescent would experience repeat pregnancies.[40,42] This lack of educational achievement in adolescent parents translates into long-term economic disadvantage with higher unemployment, less prestigious jobs, and lower incomes as adults.

Adolescent fathers and the families of adolescent parents are also likely to be under a great deal of stress.[38,43] Pressures from family and peer groups, and an inability to cope with perceived responsibilities, whether he is married or not, may make the adolescent father less likely to succeed in educational and vocational endeavors.

Since the adolescent mother has not finished her own psychologic and educational development, and is often faced with a variety of socioeconomic problems, it is not surprising that she may have difficulty coping with the emotional and physical needs of her child. While there may be no clear indication that children of adolescent parents are more frequently victims of child abuse, they may be at greater risk for neglect.[43] Children of adolescent parents are at increased risk of dying from sudden infant death syndrome (SIDS),[32,44,45] have reduced growth parameters (weight and height),[46] lower intelligence quotients,[46,47] and poor school performances.[48] Studies of younger mothers have suggested poorer child-rearing practices.[46,49]

PREVENTION OF ADOLESCENT PREGNANCY

Zelnick and Kantner[50] found that sexual intercourse among never-married teenagers increased by 30% between 1971 and 1976. Other countries with similar or even higher rates of teenage sexual activity, however, do not have adolescent pregnancy rates as high as those in the United States.[2] In these countries, it appears that better knowledge of sexuality and greater availability of contraceptive services are the most important factor in preventing pregnancy in these sexually active teenagers.

There is no ideal contraceptive method for the developing adolescent. Birth control pills, the most frequently used contraceptive among teenagers, require a methodic compliance on a daily basis for successful use. Diaphragms and other barrier methods require premeditated planning that is often lacking in adolescents' sexual behavior.[51] The intrauterine device (IUD) is associated with a three- to ninefold increase in pelvic infections.[52] The risk of infection along with other complications of insertion, expulsion, and accidental pregnancy, has led to a much more limited recommendation for use of the IUD in the adolescent. Other methods of contraception, such as periods of abstinence (rhythm method), coitus interruptus, and postcoital douching, are much less likely to be effective. It is particularly discouraging that even though adolescents today are more likely to use an effective contraception, it is uncommon for contraception to be used in a first sexual exposure, and often contraception is not used until a pregnancy has occurred.

Edwards and associates[53] have reported an encouraging sign for improved teenage pregnancy prevention. They showed a 40% decline in pregnancies over a 3-year period, when contraceptive services were provided as part of a comprehensive high-school-based health care clinic. The importance of true accessability and availability of contraceptive services cannot be overemphasized.

Approximately one-third of the nearly 1,000,000 teenagers who become pregnant each year seek pregnancy termination.[54] Often the choice between having an abortion or delivering an infant is based on particular circumstances and not necessarily on specific characteristics of the young woman herself.[55] The medical, ethical, and psychosocial issues involved in an adolescent's consideration of the alternatives of parenting, adoption, or abortion are complex. It is imperative that each pregnant teenager receive professional counseling to enable her to make an informed decision regarding these options.

IMPROVING OUTCOME OF ADOLESCENT PREGNANCY

Since the mid-1960s, when the particular problems of teenage pregnancy were first recognized, comprehensive programs for pregnant adolescents have been initiated at many medical centers.[56–60] Many of the studies on adolescent pregnancy outcome have come from these programs. The relatively favorable results may reflect the importance of this specialized approach to the adolescent. Although it may be impossible to prove which particular aspects of these programs have accounted for favorable outcomes, it appears that a comprehensive approach, including early involvement of the pregnant teenager in prenatal care, a team approach, proper nutrition counseling, and broad-based health education and counseling, is essential for success. Early prenatal care is probably the single-most-important aspect for favorable pregnancy outcome. Early prenatal care is essential for establishing dating parameters accurately, identifying health problems that may be amenable to correction, and providing time for teaching good health, hygiene, and nutrition practices. Detection and treatment of sexually transmitted diseases, urinary tract infection, anemia, and drug abuse problems are all important in lowering risk. Teenagers who receive little or no prenatal care are frequently at highest risk.[33]

A team approach is necessary to meet the multiple and complex needs of the pregnant adolescent. A staff nurse, specializing in the adolescent pregnancy program, can provide for continuity of care. Certified nurse midwives (CNMs), trained in the complex medical and psychosocial needs of the pregnant adolescent, can best act as their primary care provider, including managing normal prenatal care, labor, and delivery. The medical staff can best function as consultants should high-risk obstetrical or medical problems arise. Nurse midwives, in addition to providing preventive health teaching and guidance, serve as excellent role models for pregnant adolescents in the midst of their own psychologic development.

Nutritional assessment and counseling are essential. Nutritional assessment involves evaluation of prepregnancy weight and nutritional status, and adequacy of the present pregnancy diet. Counseling should take into consideration the continued growth requirements of the adolescent herself and also the particular social situation and ethnic background of each individual to assure the greatest chance for compliance. Teenagers with financial need should be enrolled in the local Special Supplemental Food Program for

Women, Infants, and Children (WIC Program). Counseling is also required relative to the adverse effects of smoking, alcohol, and substance abuse. The concern for good pregnancy outcome may be a significant motivational factor to allow success in eliminating these hazards.

Community health nurses and family counselors are valuable resources for pregnant adolescents and their families. These health care professionals require special training in pregnancy health education and counseling oriented toward the ethnic and social background of the community they serve. Bilingual skills, for example, may be necessary. The community health nurse and family counselor should involve the pregnant adolescent's family, as well as the adolescent father, so they may become support persons for the adolescent's prenatal care, labor, and delivery.

Health education and counseling should not be limited to pregnancy, labor, and delivery but should also include the postpartum period, basic mothering skills, and breast-feeding, child care, and contraception. This can often be most effectively accomplished in a group setting where adolescents can interact with their peers.

A social service contact should be made for each pregnant adolescent and her family. Behavioral, social, and economic assessments and intervention are frequently required. Linkages with a variety of social, governmental, religious, and educational agencies facilitate the care and support of the pregnant adolescent. In addition to supervising and guiding family counselors, social workers will also need to intervene in situations of potential abuse, drug addiction, and lack of financial or family support resources. Adolescents desiring adoption for their babies should be handled through licensed professional agencies.

A comprehensive adolescent pregnancy program, as described above, had been established at our Prenatal Clinic at Baystate Medical Center in Springfield, Massachusetts. In 1983, there were 217 deliveries, including 23 deliveries to mothers 15 years old or younger. Outcome data from the Adolescent Pregnancy Clinic revealed a low birth weight rate of 8.75%, lower than that of our overall clinic rate. A continuing problem, however, has been late registration in the Adolescent Pregnancy Clinic. First trimester pregnancy registrants has been only 27%, while third-trimester registration has not been lower than 20%. The key to obtaining early prenatal care and compliance appears to be direct community outreach efforts and specific attention to the special needs of the individual adolescent.

Comprehensive adolescent pregnancy programs should provide obstetric, nutritional, and psychosocial counseling services in a single setting. With adequate attention to the socioeconomic, nutritional, and psychosocial needs of the adolescent, a comprehensive adolescent pregnancy program should result in favorable pregnancy outcome for both mother and infant. However, the long-term solution to the adolescent pregnancy problem should be prevention. From an analysis of determinants of teenage pregnancy in other developed countries, success has occurred when pregnancy, rather than adolescent sexual activity, is identified as the major problem.[2] Comprehensive sex education programs in the public school systems and an increased availability of contraceptive services to all teenagers appear to be the primary means of further lowering the rate of adolescent pregnancy.

REFERENCES

1. National Center for Health Statistics: Advance Report of Final Natality Statistics, 1981. Vital Health Stat Rep 1983;32 (suppl).
2. Jones EF, Forrest JD, Goldman N, et al: Teenage pregnancy in developed countries: Determinants and policy implications. Fam Plann Perspect 1985;17:53.
3. Battaglia FC, Frazier TM, Hellegers AE: Obstetric and pediatric complications of juvenile pregnancy. Pediatrics 1963;32:902.
4. Hulka JF, Schaaf JT: Obstetrics in adolescents: A controlled study of deliveries by mothers 15 years of age and under. Obstet Gynecol 1964;23:678.
5. Shapiro S, Schlesinger ER, Newbitt REL: Infant, perinatal, maternal and childhood mortality in the United States. Cambridge, MA, Harvard University Press, 1968:56–64.
6. Dwyer JF: Teenage pregnancy. Am J Obstet Gynecol 1974;118:373.
7. Duenhoelter JM, Jiminez JM, Baumann G: Pregnancy performance of patients under fifteen years of age. Obstet Gynecol 1975;46:49.
8. Jekel JF, Harrison JT, Bancroft DRE, et al: A comparison of the health index and subsequent babies born to school age mothers. Am J Public Health 1975;65:370.
9. Fielding J: Adolescent pregnancy revisited. New Engl J Med 1978;299:893.
10. Spellacy W, Mahan C, Cruz A: The adolescent's first pregnancy: a controlled study. South Med J 1978;71:768.
11. Hayes L, Crovitz E: Adolescent pregnancy. South Med J 1979;31:869.
12. Baldwin W: Adolescent pregnancy and childbearing—an overview. Semin Perinatol 1981;5:1.
13. Zlatnik F, Burmeister L: Low gynecologic age: An obstetric risk factor. Am J Obstet Gynecol 1967;128:183.
14. Erkan K, Rimer B, Stine O: Juvenile pregnancy: Role of physiologic maturity. Md Med J 1971;20:50.
15. Sherline DM: When the mother is a child herself. Contemp OB/GYN 1984;24:83.
16. Moerman ML: Growth of the birth canal in adolescent girls. Am J Obstet Gynecol 1982;143:528.
17. Hassan HM, Falls FJ: The young primipara. Am J Obstet Gynecol 1964;58:256.
18. Marchetti AA, Menaker JS: Pregnancy and the adolescent. Am J Obstet Gynecol 1950;59:1013.
19. Bochner K: Pregnancies in juveniles. Am J Obstet Gynecol 1962;83:269.
20. Sherline DM, Arnolds CW: Obstetrics and medical risk of adolescent pregnancy. Trans Am Gynecol Obstet Soc 1983;1:33.
21. Menken J: The health and demographic consequences of adolescent pregnancy and childbearing. In: Chilman, CS, ed. Adolescent pregnancy and childbearing: Findings from research. Washington, DC; U.S. Department of Health and Human Services, U.S. Government Printing Office, 1980:151–205.
22. Osofsky MJ: Mitigating the adverse affects of early parenthood. Contemp OB/GYN 1985;25:57.
23. Carey WM, McCann-Sanford T, Davidson EC Jr: Adolescent age and obstetrical risk. Semin Perinatol 1981;5:9.

24. Pritchard JA, MacDonald PC, Gant NF: Williams obstetrics, 17th ed. Norwalk, CT: Appleton-Century-Crofts, 1985:525–560.
25. Feeney JG, Scott JS: Pre-eclampsia and changed paternity. Eur J Obstet Gynecol Reprod Biol 1980;11:35.
26. McCormick MC, Shapiro S, Starfield B: High risk young mothers: Infant mortality and morbidity in four areas in the United States, 1973–1978. Am J Public Health 1984;74:18.
27. Zuckerman B, Alpert JJ, Dooling E, et al: Neonatal outcome: is adolescent pregnancy a risk factor? Pediatrics 1983;71:489.
28. James W: Newer approaches in the management of the pregnant unmarried adolescent. J Natl Med Assoc 1972;64:483.
29. Wiener G, Milton T: Demographic correlates of low birth weight. Am J Epidemiol 1970;91:260.
30. Zakler J, Andelman S, Bauer F: The young adolescent as an obstetric risk. Am J Obstet Gynecol 1969;103:305.
31. Miller HC, Merritt TA: Fetal growth in humans. Chicago: Yearbook Medical Publishers, 1979:91–98.
32. Merritt TA, Lawrence RA, Naeye RL: The infants of adolescent mothers. Pediatr Ann 1980;9:100.
33. Elster AB: The effect of maternal age, parity, and prenatal care on perinatal outcome in adolescent mothers. Am J Obstet Gynecol 1984;169:845.
34. Dott A, Fort A: Medical and social factors affecting early teenage pregnancy: a literature review and summary of the findings of the Louisiana Infant Mortality Study. Am J Obstet Gynecol 1976;125:532.
35. Niswander NR, Gordon M: The women and their pregnancies. Philadelphia: WB Saunders, 1972:213–219.
36. Lawrence RA, Merritt TA: Infants of adolescent mothers: perinatal, neonatal and infancy outcome. Semin Perinatol 1981;5:19.
37. Shapiro S, McCormick MC, Starfield B, et al: Relevance of correlates of infant deaths for significant mortality at 1 year of age. Am J Obstet Gynecol 1980;136:363.
38. McAnarney ER, Thiede HA: Adolescent pregnancy and childbearing: what we have learned in a decade and what remains to be learned. Semin Perinatol 1981;5:91.
39. Garn SM, Shaw MA, McCabe KD: Effects of socioeconomic status and race on weight-defined and gestational prematurity in the United States. In: Reed DM, Stanley FJ, eds. The epidemiology of prematurity. Baltimore, Munich: Urban and Schwarzenberg, 1977:127–143.
40. Furstenberg F: The social consequences of teenage parenthood. Fam Plann Perspect 1976;8:148.
41. Card J, Wise L: Teenage mothers and teenage fathers: The impact of early childbearing on the parents' personal and professional lives. Fam Plann Perspect 1978; 10:199.
42. Klerman L, Jekel J: School-age mothers: Problems, programs, and policy. Hamden, CT: The Shoe String Press, 1973.
43. Elster AB, McAnarney ER: Medical and psychosocial risks of pregnancy and childbearing during adolescence. Pediatr Ann 1980;9:84.
44. Bergman AB, Ray CG, Pomeroy MA, et al: Studies of the sudden infant death syndrome in King County, Washington. III: Epidemiology. Pediatrics 1972;49:860.
45. Kraus JF, Franti CE, Borhani NO: Discriminatory risk factors in postneonatal sudden unexplained death. Am J Epidemiol 1972;96:328.
46. Oppel WC, Royston AB: Teenage births: some social, psychological and physical sequellae. Am J Public Health 1971;61:751.
47. Lobl M, Welcher DW, Mellits ED: Maternal age and intellectual functioning of offspring. Johns Hopkins Med J 1971;128:347.
48. Hardy JB, Welcher DW, Stanley J, et al: Long-range outcome of adolescent pregnancy. Clin Obstet Gynecol 1978;21:1217.

49. Williams TM: Childrearing practices of young mothers: What we know, how it matters, why it's so little. Am J Orthopsychiatry 1974;44:70.

50. Zelnik M, Kantner JF: Sexual and contraceptive experience of young unmarried women in the United States, 1976 and 1971. Fam Plann Perspect 1977;9:55.

51. Zelnik M, Kantner JF: Reasons for non-use of contraception by sexually active women aged 15–19. Fam Plann Perspect 1979;11:289.

52. Greydanus DE: Alternatives to adolescent pregnancy: A discussion of contraceptive literature from 1960 to 1980. Semin Perinatol 1981;5:53.

53. Edwards LE, Steinman ME, Arnold KA, et al: Adolescent pregnancy preventive services in high school clinics. Fam Plann Perspect 1980;12:6.

54. National Center for Health Statistics: Natality Statistics from the National Center for Health Statistics. Vital Health Stat Rep 1979;27 (suppl).

55. Bracken MB, Klarimen LV, Bracken M: Abortion, adoption or motherhood: an empirical study of decision making during pregnancy. Am J Obstet Gynecol 1978;130:251.

56. Sarrel PM: The university hospital and the teenage, unwed mother. Am J Obstet Gynecol 1967;57:1308.

57. Osofsky JH, Hagen JH, Wood PW: A program for pregnant school girls. AM J Obstet Gynecol 1968;100:1026.

58. Klein L: Early teenage pregnancy, contraception, and repeat pregnancy. Am J Obstet Gynecol 1974;120:249.

59. McAnarney ER, Adams BN: Development of an adolescent maternity project in Rochester, New York. Public Health Rep 1977;92:154.

60. Youngs DD, Neibyl JR, Blake DA, Shipp DA, King RM: Understanding adolescent pregnancy. In: Youngs DD, Ehrhardt AA, eds. Psychosomatic obstetrics and gynecology. New York: Appleton-Century Crofts, 1980:199–210.

CHAPTER 7

Ultrasound of the Pediatric and Adolescent Patient

Jane Share, MD, and Rita Teele, MD

This chapter considers those clinical problems in adolescent gynecology for which ultrasonography is a diagnostic aid. Ultrasonography should not be used in the place of a pelvic examination unless the examination is technically difficult or is refused by the patient. Ultrasonograms do not provide pathologic information directly; they are black-and-white representations of anatomy and must be evaluated and correlated with the clinical findings. Nowhere has ultrasonography been as valuable as in the field of obstetrics and gynecology, but its increased use has also shown its limitations.

PREPARATION AND TECHNIQUE

The ultrasonographic examination is performed with the patient supine. Her bladder should be fully distended to provide an "acoustic window" for the ultrasonic beam. This usually can be accomplished by having the patient drink several glasses of water an hour or two before the examination.

The pelvis is scanned in the transverse and longitudinal planes to define fully the anatomy of the uterus and adnexae. Because of the association of uterine and renal anomalies, views of the kidneys should be included as part of the examination.

NORMAL ANATOMY

The uterus should be identified throughout childhood. The prepubertal uterus measures 2–3.3 cm in length and .5–1 cm in width.[1] The fundus is about the same size as the cervix (Figure 7-1A). With the onset of puberty,

Clinical Practice of Gynecology: **3,** 72–92, 1989
© 1989 Elsevier Science Publishing Co., Inc.
655 Avenue of the Americas, New York, NY 10010
ISSN 1043-3198/89/$3.50

the uterine fundus enlarges. The average postpubertal uterus measures from 5 to 8 cm in length; the fundus is from 1.6 to 3 cm in width (Figure 7-1B).[1]

Ovaries are generally less than 1 cm³ in volume in the prepubertal age group (.13–.9 cm³). The normal adolescent has mean ovarian volumes of 4 cm³ (1.8–5.7 cm³).[1] Follicular cysts up to 3 cm in size may be seen in the ovary near the time of ovulation and are normal (Figure 7-1C).[2]

USES OF ULTRASONOGRAPHY

Primary Amenorrhea

The major role for ultrasonography in an adolescent with primary amenorrhea is to document anatomy—to determine whether or not ovaries and the uterus are present and normal in appearance.

Gonadal dysgenesis accounts for 10–25% of all cases of primary amenorrhea.[3] Most of the patients with gonadal dysgenesis have an abnormality of the sex chromosomes but some have a normal karyotype. Of those pa-

FIGURE 7-1 Normal uterus and ovary. (A) Longitudinal scan of a normal prepubertal uterus (arrows). The fundus and cervix are about the same size. (B) Longitudinal scan of a normal postpubertal uterus. With puberty, the fundus assumes a bulbous configuration and is larger than the cervix. (C) Longitudinal scan of a postpubertal ovary containing a small follicular cyst (arrow). Although in young girls the ovaries may not be well outlined on ultrasonograms, the adolescent's ovary should always be visualized with good ultrasonographic technique.

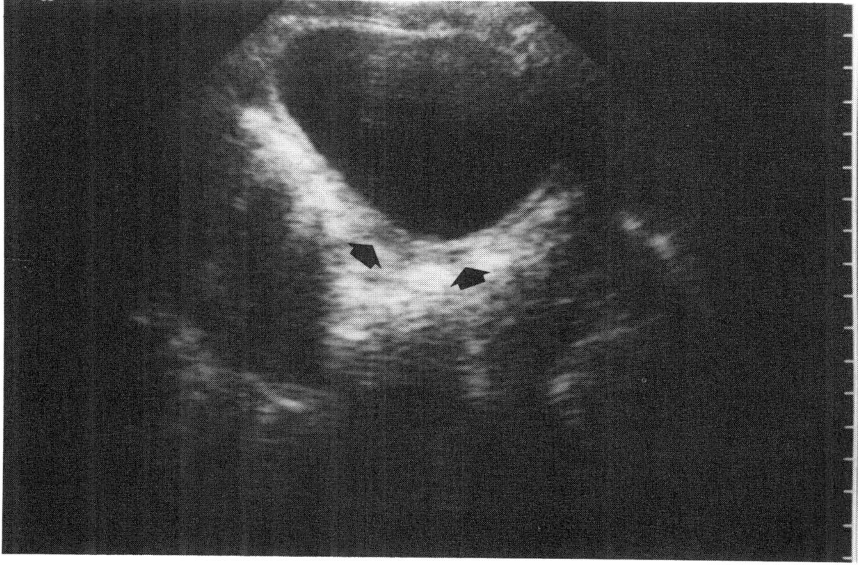

A

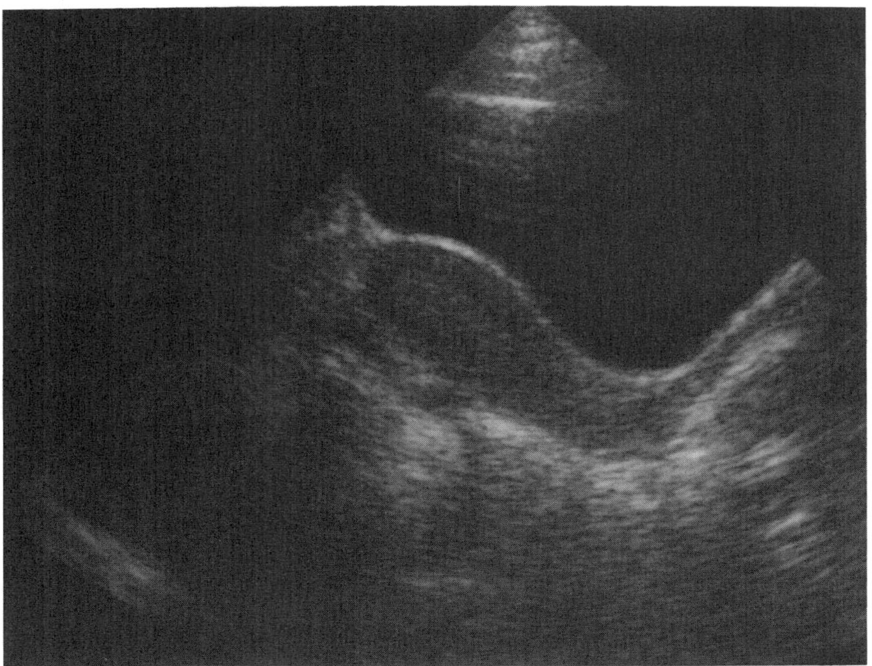

B

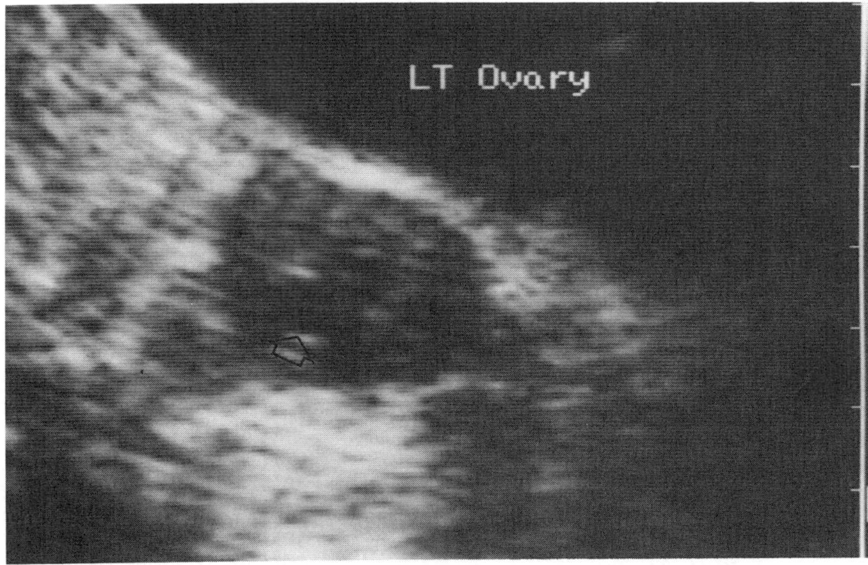

C
FIGURE 7-1 (*continued*)

tients with a chromosomal defect, about one-half are 45X; the rest have a variety of other abnormalities of the X chromosome.[4]

Ultrasonography in patients with the 45X karyotype, or "classic" Turner's syndrome, usually reveals absent ovaries and a uterus of prepubertal size (see Figure 7-3). Ultrasonograms in patients who have chromosomal mosaicism or other of the X chromosome alterations are variably abnormal. The ovaries may be nonvisible, small, or appear normal. Likewise, the uterus ranges in size from prepubertal to normal adult.[5]

Because of an increased incidence of renal anomalies associated with gonadal dysgenesis, the kidneys in affected individuals should be studied at the time of ultrasonography. Horseshoe kidney, ureteropelvic junction obstruction, and ectopic kidney are some of the abnormalities encountered.[6]

Individuals with pure gonadal dysgenesis are those with primary amenorrhea and absent secondary sexual characteristics associated with a normal karyotype. These patients typically have streak gonads (virtually never identified on ultrasonography) and an infantile uterus.[7]

Absence of the uterus as a cause of primary amenorrhea is uncommon. The Mayer–Rokitansky–Kuster–Hauser syndrome and the testicular feminization syndrome are the two major syndromes in this category. Although rare, the Mayer–Rokitansky–Kuster–Hauser syndrome is the second-most common cause of primary amenorrhea following gonadal dysgenesis. The ovaries are normal. Congenital absence of the vagina and an absent or abnormal uterus are part of the syndrome, which is due to abnormal development of Mullerian duct derivatives. The range of uterine abnormalities, including agenesis, hypoplasia, and duplication—with or without obstruction—can be demonstrated with ultrasonography (Figure 7-2A). Because of time-related embryologic development, the kidneys and skeleton are affected in 50% and 12% of cases, respectively. Renal abnormalities include unilateral agenesis, horseshoe kidney, and crossed fused ectopia (Figure 7-2B). The majority of skeletal abnormalities involve the spine and include abnormalities of segmentation, rudimentary, and wedge vertebrae.[8]

Patients with the testicular feminization syndrome are genotypically male (XY) but phenotypically female because of end-organ insensitivity to testosterone. They have neither uterus nor ovaries. Intraabdominal testes are present and may sometimes be visualized on ultrasonography as unusual soft tissue densities in the "adnexal" regions behind the bladder.[9]

An increasing number of girls with primary amenorrhea are survivors of childhood malignancy that have been treated with radiotherapy and/or chemotherapy. Both agents affect the reproductive system. Ovarian failure occurs in most patients after a single dose to the pelvis from 650 to 750 rad or a fractionated dose from 1,500 to 2,500 rad.[10] Arrest of uterine growth may result as a direct effect of radiotherapy in childhood. Uterine hypoplasia from lack of stimulation from the ovaries is an indirect result of pelvic irradiation (Figure 7-3).

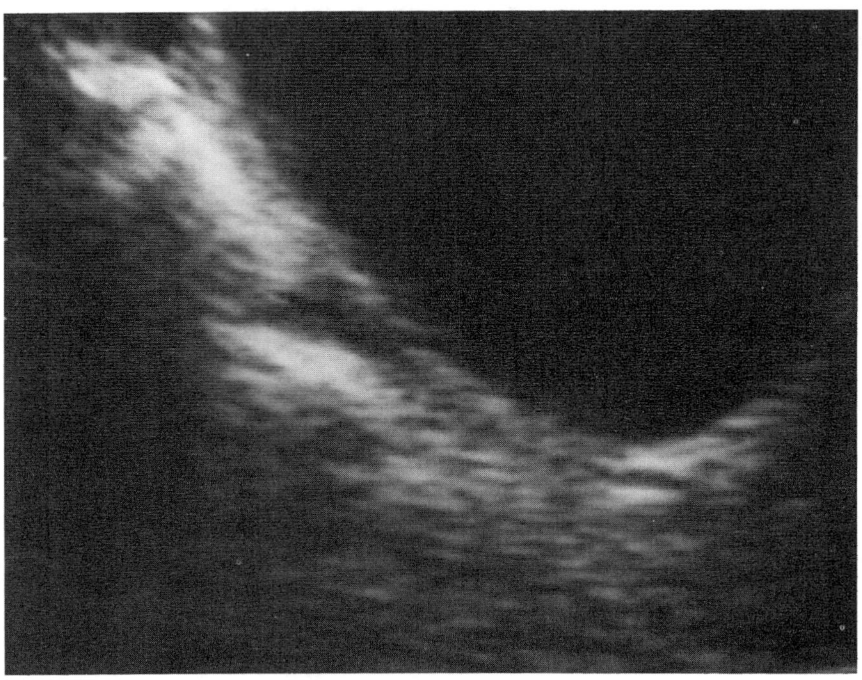

A

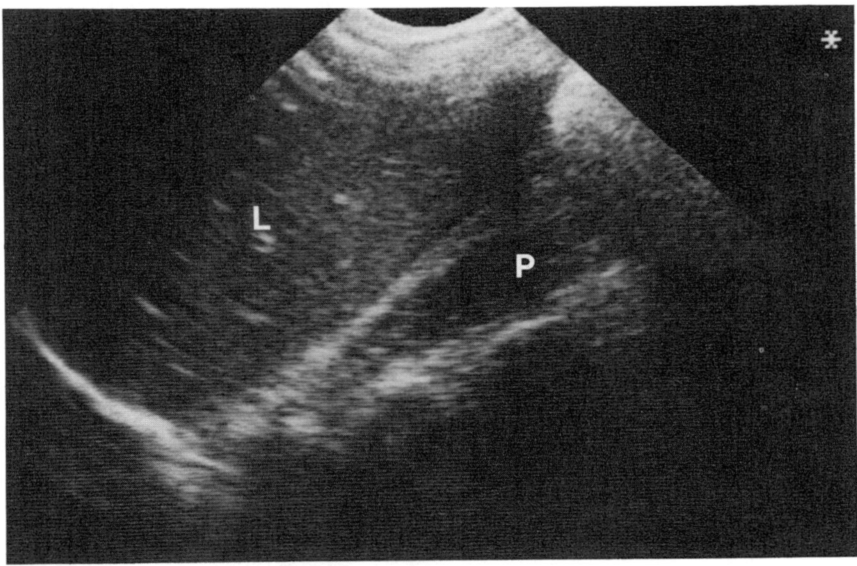

B

FIGURE 7-2 Vaginal agenesis with solitary left kidney. (A) Absent uterus. Midline longitudinal scan through a distended urinary bladder. No uterus is seen. (B) Absent right kidney. Longitudinal scan of the right upper quadrant shows only liver and psoas, and an empty renal fossa (L, liver; P, psoas). The left kidney was normal. The patient was a normally developed 16-year-old female (46XX) with primary amenorrhea. She later underwent vaginoplasty.

An infrequent cause of primary amenorrhea associated with a small uterus is Kallman's syndrome, which is rare and characterized by sexual infantilism and anosmia. It is caused by complete or partial agenesis of the olfactory bulbs and abnormalities in the hypothalamus.[11]

Secondary Amenorrhea

Pregnancy is the major cause of secondary amenorrhea. Ultrasonography is not advocated as a means of diagnosing pregnancy. A human chorionic gonadotropin (HCG) level should be obtained prior to the ultrasonogram in a patient suspected of being pregnant; an intrauterine gestational sac will

FIGURE 7-3 Hypoplastic uterus. Longitudinal midline scan shows a uterus of prepubertal size and shape in this 15-year-old girl with primary amenorrhea. She had received pelvic irradiation at age 1 year 3 months for a pelvic neuroblastoma. Other causes for uterine hypoplasia such as gonadal dysgenesis would look the same.

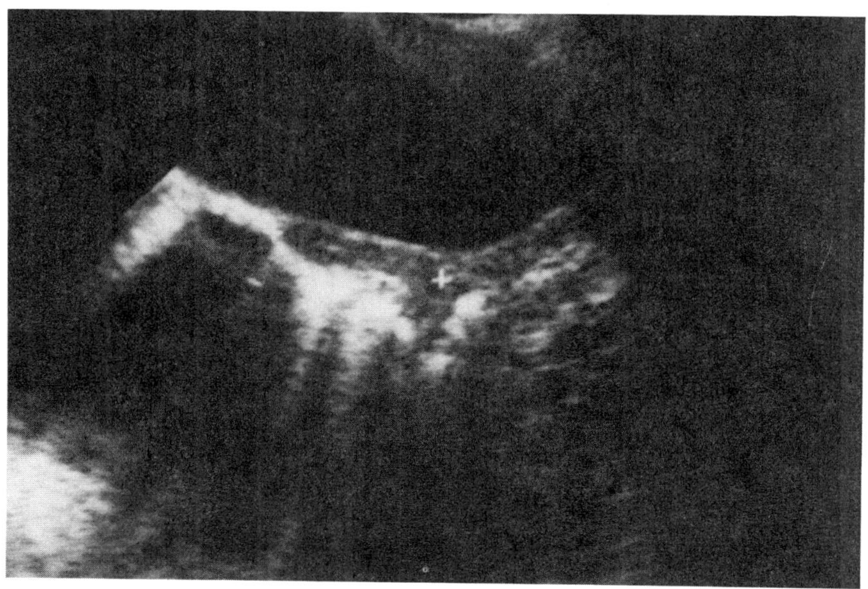

not be visible on transabdominal scans in a normal pregnancy until the HCG is >6,500 mIU/mL in plasma. (Each hospital laboratory should provide data on units used for HCG testing. The current literature comparing ultrasonographic findings and HCG values is confusing because different units have been used and reported by various groups.)

Endovaginal ultrasonography, a relatively new technique, is now being used in the evaluation of early pregnancy. This method of imaging is not hindered by patient obesity and does not require a full urinary bladder. Compared with a transabdominal examination, endovaginal ultrasonography is often more sensitive in the evaluation of normal intrauterine pregnancy, ectopic pregnancy, and spontaneous incomplete abortion.[12] This technique probably will play an expanding role in the evaluation of complicated early pregnancies, especially when transabdominal ultrasonography is difficult to perform or evaluate.

Because adolescents have a high incidence of pre- and postnatal problems compared to the older population, we feel that they should be evaluated by ultrasonographers with expertise in fetal and obstetric disorders if the pregnancy is to be carried to term.

Approximately 50% of patients with polycystic ovarian disease (PCO) experience amenorrhea.[13] This syndrome has outgrown the classic definition of oligomenorrhea, obesity, and hirsutism associated with very large ovaries as described by Stein and Leventhal. Patients with PCO may have hyperandrogenism and ovaries that are normal in size or slightly enlarged. Others have polycystic ovaries without signs of hyperandrogenism.[14]

Ultrasonography shows enlarged ovaries in about 70% of patients with PCO; the remaining ovaries are normal in size (Figure 7-4).[15,16] Ultrasonographic visualization of increased numbers of developing follicles has also been reported in polycystic ovaries.[16]

Ovarian tumors of all types occur with increased frequency in patients with PCO; the incidence ranges from 4.6% to 20%.[17] Ultrasonography should be helpful in screening for this complication of the disease.

Symptoms of secondary amenorrhea can be caused by both masculinizing and feminizing ovarian tumors. Occasionally, other ovarian tumors, such as cystadenoma, cystadenofibroma, and dysgerminoma, are hormonally active and cause secondary amenorrhea.[3]

Pelvic Mass/Pelvic Pain

Ultrasonograms in patients with pelvic pain and no palpable pelvic mass often result in little useful diagnostic information. Causes for pelvic pain include Mittelschmerz, pelvic inflammatory disease, and endometriosis. Pain is often a presenting symptom in patients with a pelvic mass, and it is the role of the ultrasonographer to characterize the mass and provide a differential diagnoses.

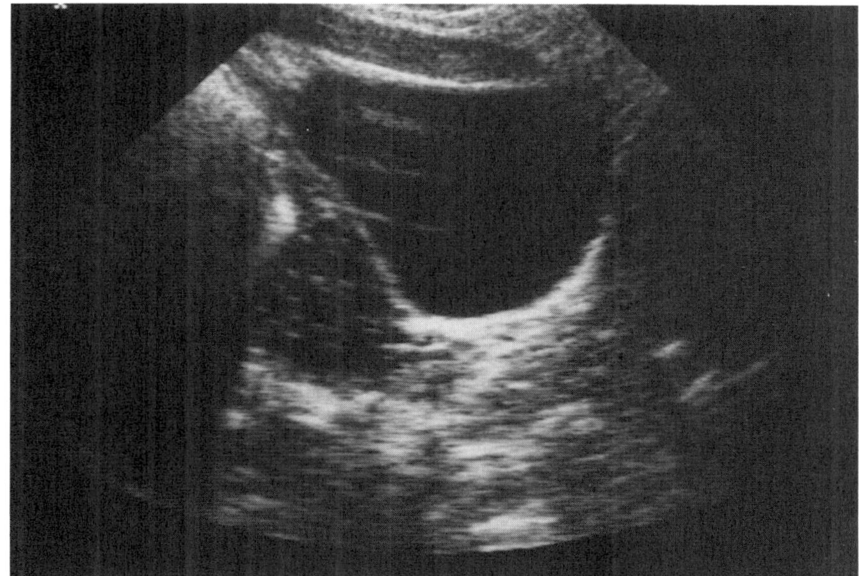

A

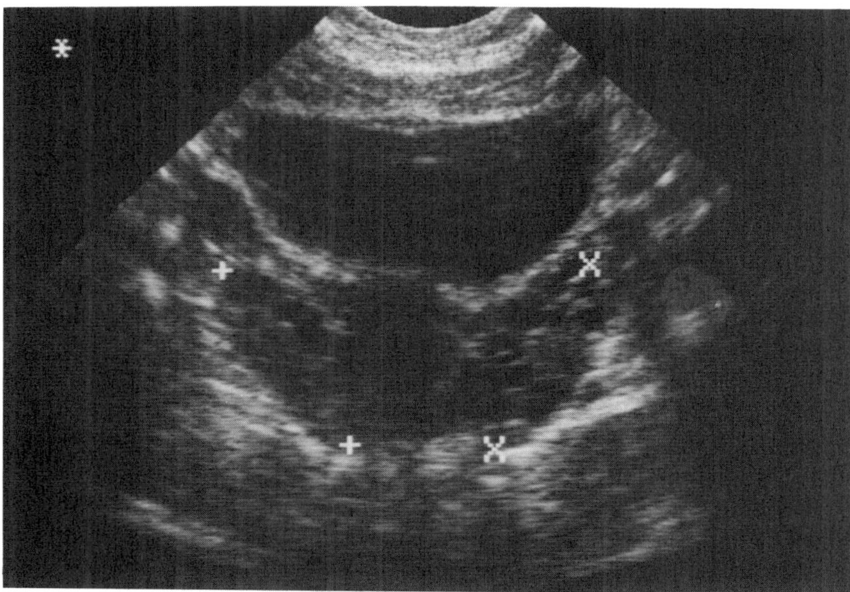

B

FIGURE 7-4 Polycystic ovarian disease. (A) Longitudinal scan of the left ovary. (B) Transverse scan of both ovaries. The ovaries are enlarged and contain multiple small cysts. The patient was a 17-year-old with pelvic pain and menstrual irregularity. Her LH/FSH ratio was greater than 3:1 (normal, about 1:1).

Ovarian Lesions

By far the most common pelvic masses in adolescent girls are ovarian in origin. Of these, simple ovarian cysts are most frequent.[18] They are typically unilocular and have no internal debris. These cysts may reach giant size, but most are 3–6 cm in diameter. Simple cysts in most cases can be managed conservatively; a repeat ultrasonogram in 2–4 weeks may show that the cyst has become smaller or disappeared. Surgery is reserved for those in whom there is persistence of a large cyst or pain, possibly related to torsion (Figure 7-5).

A septated cystic mass in the ovary is more of a diagnostic problem than a simple cyst, and the ultrasonographer is usually unable to make a specific diagnosis. A septated cystic mass has been seen in a variety of lesions, including simple cyst, cystadenofibroma, cystadenoma, and teratoma (Figure 7-6).[18] Associated ascites is a sign of ovarian tumor.

FIGURE 7-5 Simple ovarian cyst. Longitudinal midline scan shows a 7-cm cystic structure anterior to the uterus (arrow). (In this patient, the bladder was empty. Care must be taken to avoid mistaking a cyst for the bladder.) The patient was a 16-year-old with intermittent right lower quadrant pain for 3 weeks. At surgery, cyst aspiration and fenestration were performed.

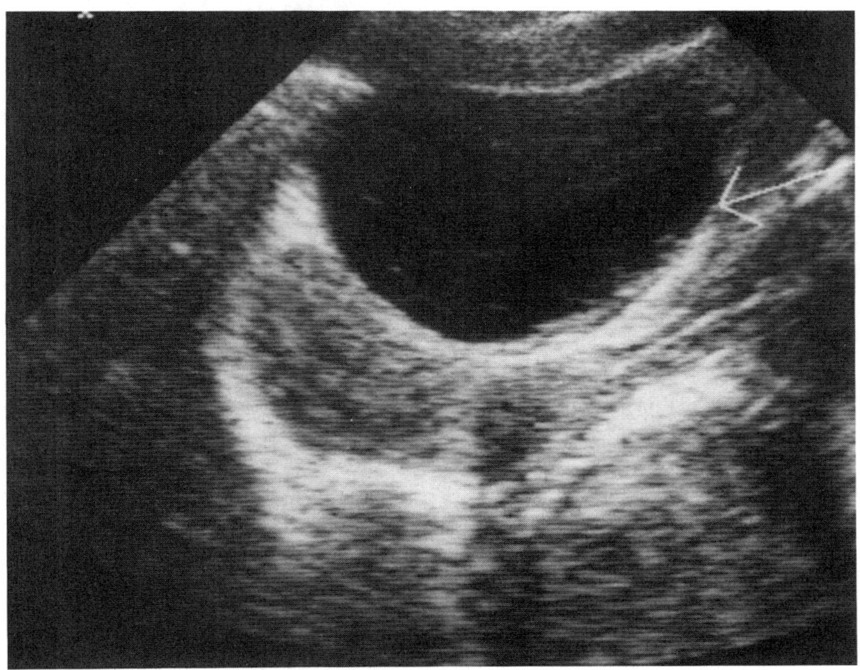

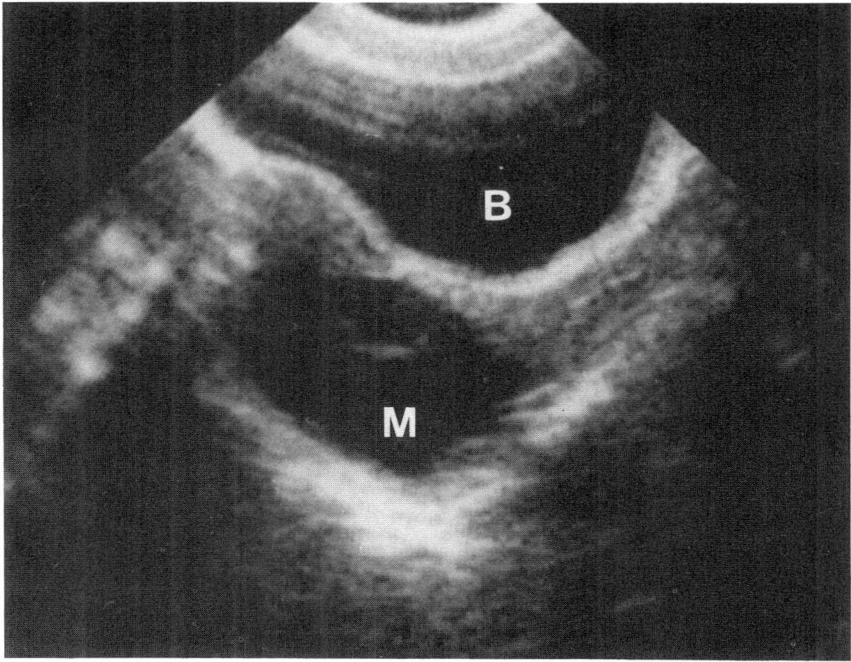

FIGURE 7-6 Mucinous cystadenoma. Longitudinal scan to the right of midline shows a loculated cystic mass (M, mass; B, bladder). This was found in an asymptomatic 20-year-old on routine physical examination. There was no way to differentiate this type of tumor (unusual in adolescents) from other cystic ovarian masses on the preoperative scans.

The differential diagnosis of solid and mixed cystic and solid adnexal masses is extensive, and it includes hemorrhage into an ovarian cyst, ovarian torsion, ovarian neoplasm, ectopic pregnancy, tubo-ovarian abscess, and periappendiceal abscess. Correlation of the ultrasonographic findings with clinical and laboratory examination is extremely important in these cases.

Bleeding into an ovarian cyst can result in a mass that appears truly solid. As the clot forms and then resorbs, the mass passes through a mixed solid/cystic phase and then becomes purely cystic. As a result the ultrasonographic findings are quite variable and fairly nonspecific. One large series reported that most hemorrhagic ovarian cysts were heterogeneous (83%); no completely anechoic lesions were found.[19] Other features of hemorrhagic ovarian cysts include a thick-rimmed mass, septations, and fluid in the cul-de-sac (Figure 7-7). If the patient with a suspected hemorrhagic ovarian cyst is stable and can be followed, a repeat ultrasonogram may show a

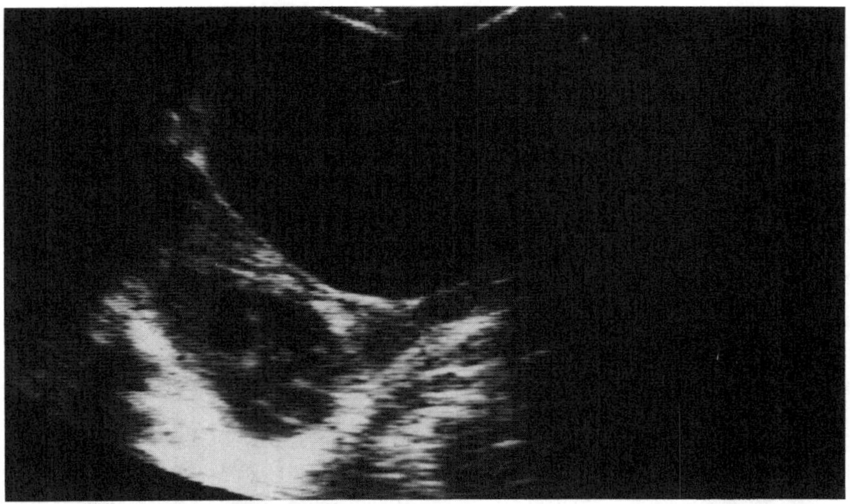

FIGURE 7-7 Hemorrhagic ovarian cyst. Longitudinal scan of the right adnexa shows a thick-walled septated cystic mass. The patient was a 15-year-old with lower abdominal pain, nausea, and vomiting.

change in the appearance of the mass, reflecting lysis of the clot, which can be helpful in establishing the diagnosis.[20]

Ovarian torsion can occur in the absence of any intrinsic adnexal abnormality. More commonly, however, there is some form of adnexal mass present, usually cystic. The torsion usually involves both the ovary and fallopian tube, and it is more common on the right than on the left. The ultrasonographic patterns in torsion are often nonspecific and include completely cystic, complex, and solid masses (Figure 7-8A).[21] A pattern consisting of a large solid mass with peripheral follicular cysts, representing the enlarged, ischemic, and hemorrhagic ovary with its peripheral cysts intact, has been described as a fairly characteristic sign of ovarian torsion (Figure 7-8B).[22] Fluid in the cul-de-sac may be associated.

FIGURE 7-8 (*right*) Ovarian torsion. (A) Longitudinal scan in the right mid abdomen demonstrates a thick-walled cyst in this 16-year-old with an 11-week intrauterine pregnancy and right-upper-quadrant pain and mass. At laporotomy, a twisted ovarian cyst was found. (B) The normal adnexa may torse as in this 9½-year-old with right-lower-quadrant pain. Longitudinal image of the right adnexa shows a well-defined, 7-cm solid mass posterior to the bladder. Small cysts in the periphery of the ovary represent the follicles.

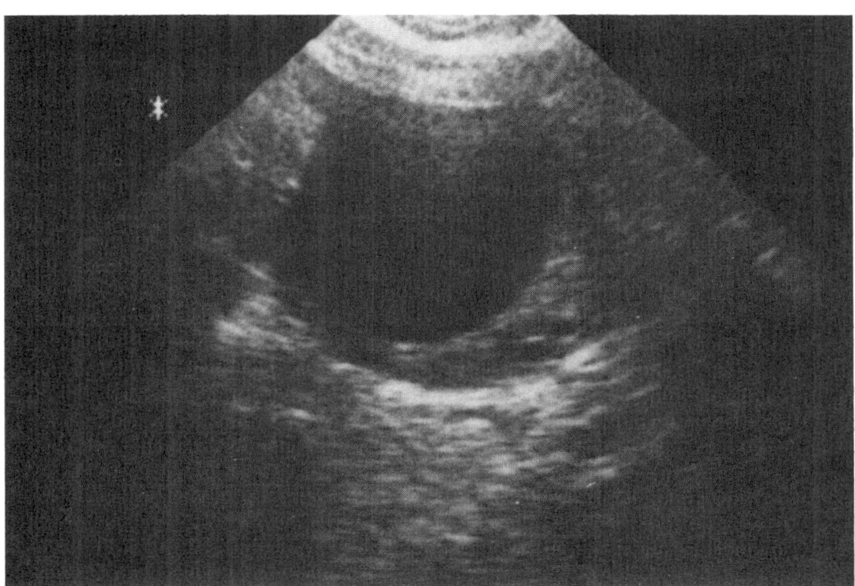

A

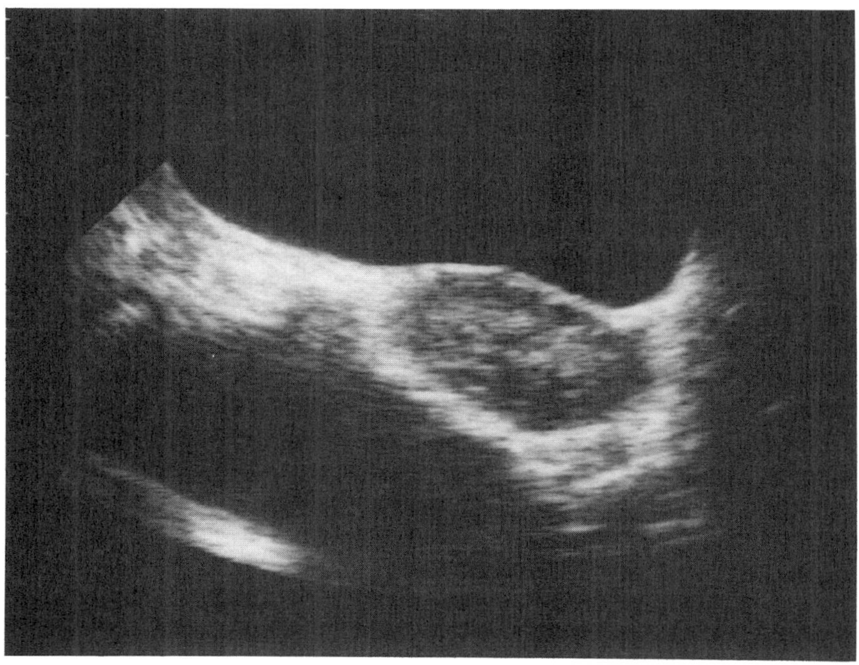

B

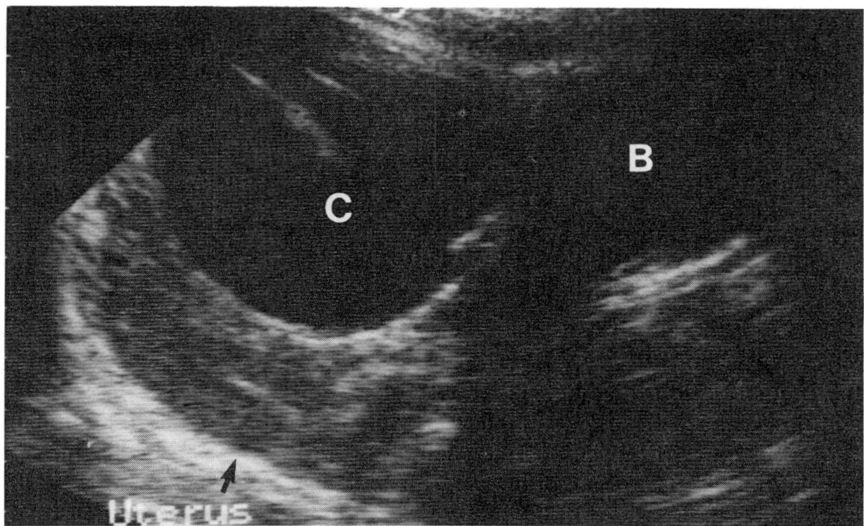

A

FIGURE 7-9 Ovarian dermoid. (A) 14-year-old patient with a 3-day history of pain and vomiting. Longitudinal midline scan shows a septated cystic mass superior to the bladder and anterior to the uterus (C, cyst; B, bladder). Because of the large cystic component, this dermoid is easily seen on the ultrasonogram. (B) 15-year-old with an asymptomatic palpable mass. This dermoid contains a large amount of fat and teeth, which cast shadows and obscure the rest of the mass. A small cystic component is present superior to the fatty portion of the lesion (m, mass; s, shadows; b, bladder). (C) An abdominal radiograph from patient B shows large lower abdominal mass (arrows). Note teeth in lower portion of mass.

The most common ovarian tumor in childhood and adolescence is a dermoid or teratoma. Most are benign; approximately 10% are bilateral.[9] Those with a cystic component are easy to demonstrate on ultrasonograms (Figure 7-9A). The fat, hair, calcifications, and occasionally teeth in a teratoma produce very reflective surfaces and cast an acoustic shadow (Figure 7-9B). If the teratoma is predominantly solid, however, it may get "lost" among bowel loops that also produce strong reflections and cast shadows. A plain film of the abdomen may help in the identification of fat, calcifications, or teeth (Figure 7-9C).

Other ovarian tumors are less common. Dysgerminomas present as a uniformly solid ovarian mass. Leukemia and lymphoma may result in diffuse enlargement of one or both ovaries. Metastatic disease involving the ovaries is extremely rare in adolescence.

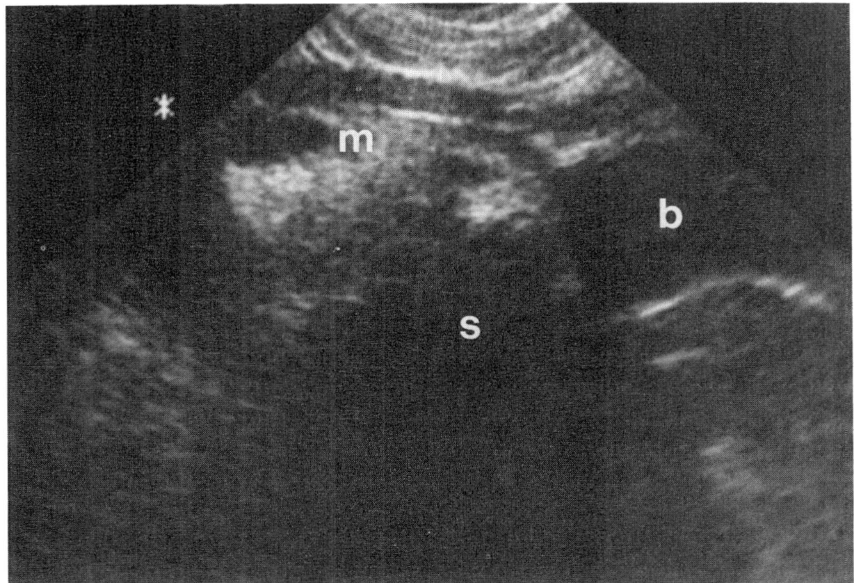

B

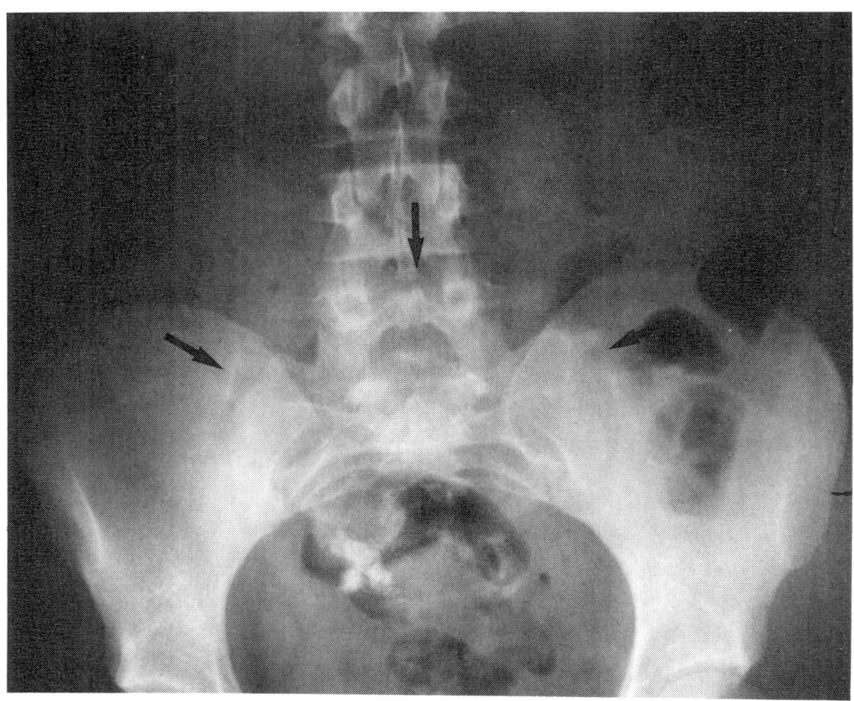

C

Pelvic Inflammatory Disease

Pelvic inflammatory disease (PID) is a frustrating entity to diagnose on ultrasonograms. It is variable in its presentation, and the sequelae of several episodes may overlap in producing anatomic changes. The ultrasonographic findings reflect the wide range of pathologic changes that may be present. Because of edema and loss of anatomic planes, a disorganized echo pattern filling the pelvis is common. Other findings include adnexal mass, unilateral or bilateral. Less commonly, isolated uterine abnormalities such as enlargement, indistinct uterine margins, and absent endometrial echoes may be seen.[23] In one prospective study, adnexal enlargement was the most useful ultrasonographic sign in differentiating adolescent patients with PID from normal controls. Uterine enlargement, fluid in the cul-de-sac, and adnexal adherence to the uterine wall were other findings that were variably present but not useful.[24]

The major differential diagnosis of acute PID in the adolescent age group is appendicitis. Short of seeing a thick-walled inflamed appendix or periappendiceal abscess, it is difficult to make the diagnosis on ultrasonography alone (Figure 7-10). An abdominal radiograph may help by showing an appendicolith in the right lower quadrant.

Ectopic Pregnancy

The diagnosis of ectopic pregnancy can be very difficult both clinically and ultrasonographically. The best evidence against an ectopic pregnancy on ultrasonograms is the presence of an intrauterine gestational sac; concomitant intrauterine and extrauterine pregnancy is extremely rare. A rarely seen *positive* sign of ectopic pregnancy is the ultrasonographic visualization of an extrauterine gestational sac containing a fetus. Usually the signs are less specific and include an adnexal mass or fluid, fluid in the cul-de-sac, uterine enlargement, and/or signs of endometrial proliferation (Figure 7-11).[25] Correlation with a test for pregnancy is mandatory.

Uterine

In the adolescent age group, uterine abnormalities less commonly than ovarian lesions cause a pelvic mass. A bicornuate uterus or a normal uterine fundus that deviates to the right or left in the pelvis may be palpated as a mass (Figure 7-12). Partial or complete duplication of the vagina with concomitant duplication of the uterus can present as a cystic pelvic mass associated with menstrual irregularity and lower abdominal pain. The mass usually represents hematocolpos in an obstructed hemivagina (Figure 7-13). Unilateral renal agenesis, usually on the side of the hematocolpos, is a common association.[26]

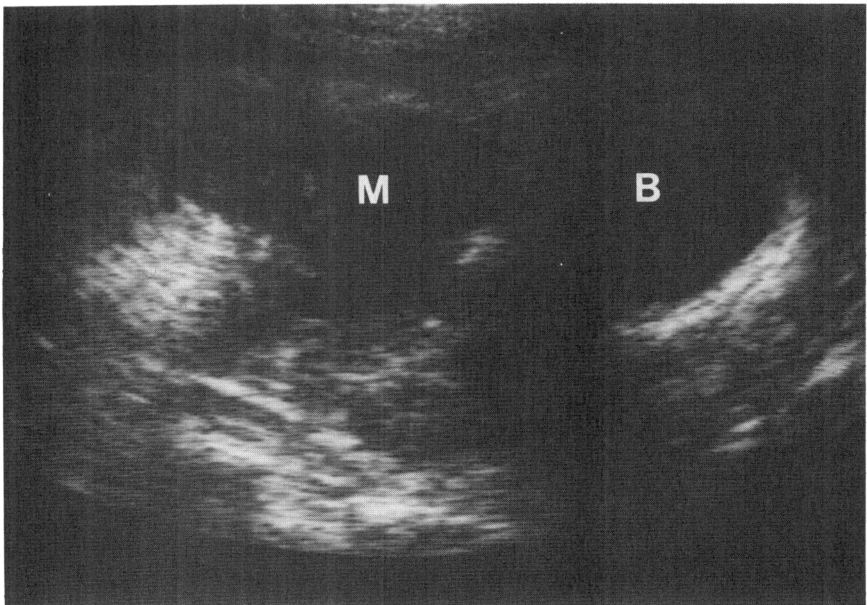

FIGURE 7-10 Periappendiceal abscess. Longitudinal scan of the right lower quadrant in this 14-year-old with pain and leukocytosis shows a septated cystic mass (M, mass; B, bladder). At surgery, a partial colectomy had to be performed when removing the abscess. There is frequently a problem differentiating pelvic inflammatory disease of gynecologic origin from appendiceal disease.

Uterine leiomyomas are unusual abnormalities in the adolescent, but when present are characterized by a pelvic mass, pain, and abnormal bleeding. They are more common in blacks and can become large at an earlier age in this group. Ultrasonographic findings include uterine enlargement and textural alteration, as well as distortion of the uterine contour (Figure 7-14).[27]

Malignant uterine tumors are rare in adolescents, but are encountered in the preadolescent.

CONCLUSION

Ultrasonography is painless, involves no irradiation, and is widely available. When used in association with a careful history and thorough physical examination, pelvic ultrasonography can be extremely useful in the management of adolescents with gynecologic problems. However, it should never be used in place of these two important clinical tools.

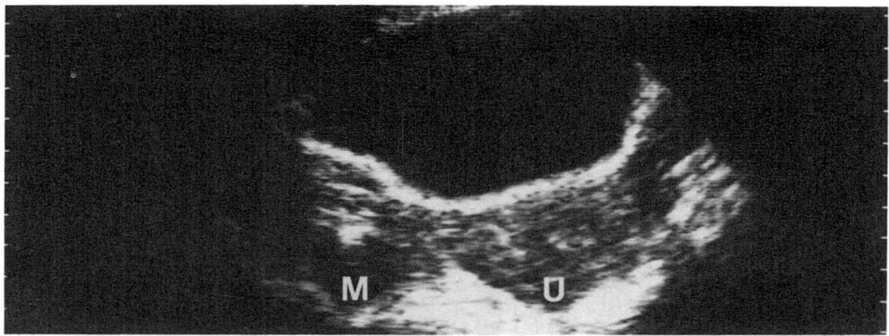

A

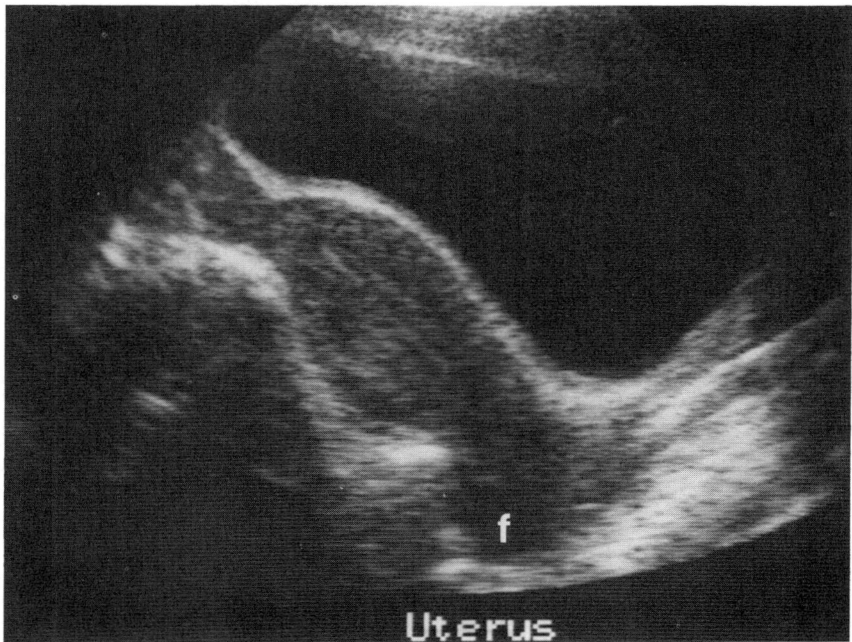

B

FIGURE 7-11 Ectopic pregnancy. (A) Transverse scan shows a complex mass in the right adnexa (M, mass; U, uterus). (B) Longitudinal midline image shows an empty uterus and free fluid in the cul-de-sac (f, fluid). The patient was a 16-year-old with a positive pregnancy test and vaginal bleeding.

FIGURE 7-12 Bicornuate uterus. (A) Axial scan of the lower uterine segment demonstrates transverse elongation of the endometrial echoes (arrows). (B) Cephalic angulation of the ultrasound beam shows divergence of the uterine fundi (arrows). There is an incidental retrouterine adnexal cyst (c, cyst).

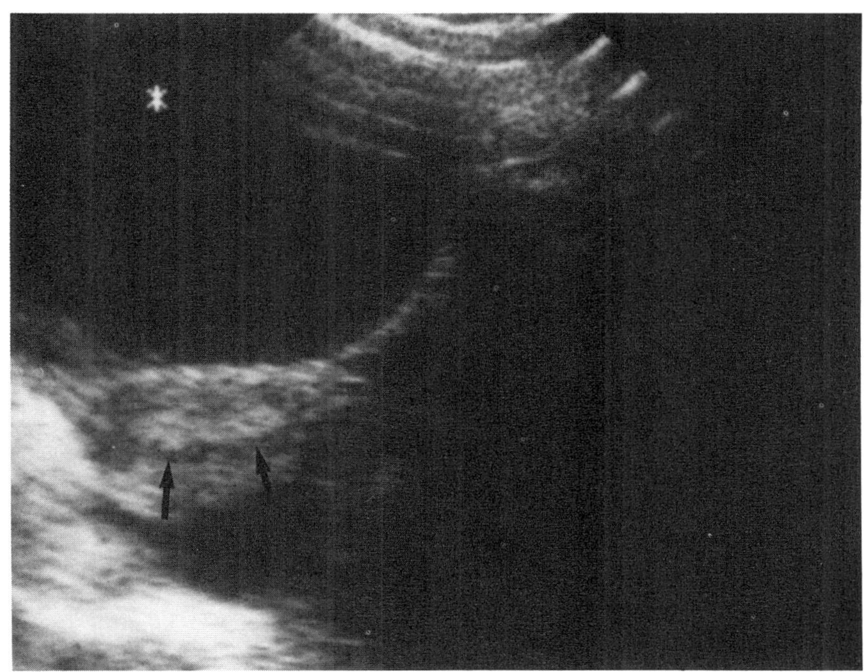

A

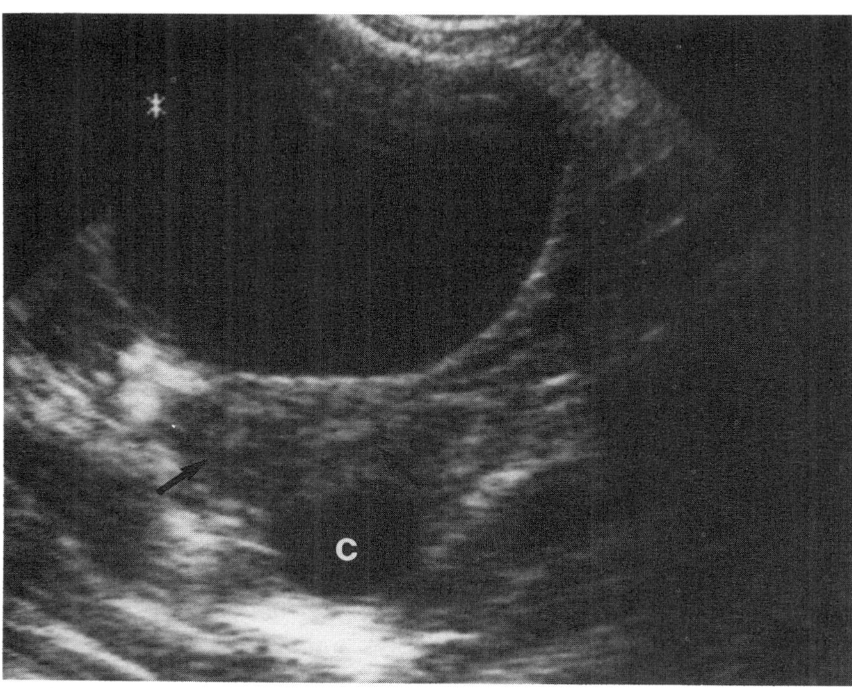

B

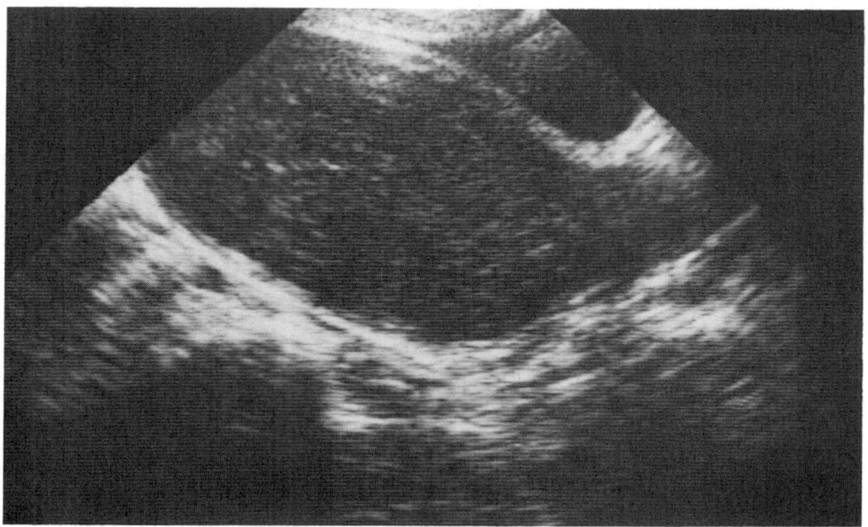

FIGURE 7-13

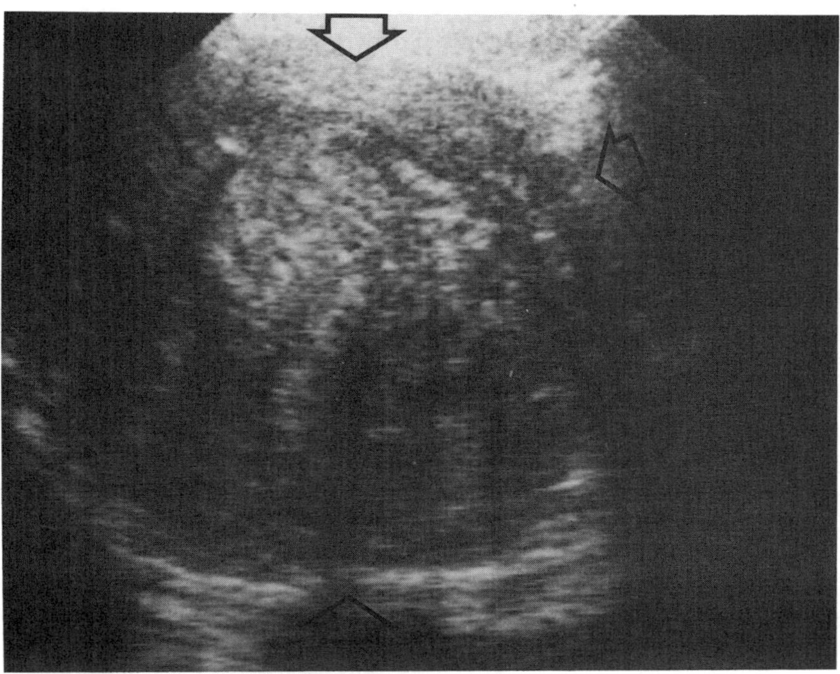

FIGURE 7-14

FIGURE 7-13 Uterine and vaginal duplication. Longitudinal scan to the left of midline shows a large pear-shaped structure containing low-level echoes. This represented hematocolpos in this 14-year-old with uterine and vaginal duplication and obstruction of the left hemivagina. There was associated left renal agenesis. At surgery, the vaginal septum was excised and 100 cc of blood evacuated.

FIGURE 7-14 Uterine leiomyoma. Longitudinal image shows a 10-cm solid mass superior to the bladder (arrows). Normal pelvic structures could not be identified with certainty. This 17-year-old presented with right lower quadrant pain for 5 days. At surgery, a myomectomy was performed for a large uterine fibroid.

REFERENCES

1. Lippe BM, Sample WF: Pelvic ultrasonography in pediatric and adolescent endocrine disorders. J Pediatr 1978;92:897.
2. Renaud RL, Macler J, Dervain I, et al: Echographic study of follicular maturation and ovulation during the normal menstrual cycle. Fertil Steril 1980;33:272.
3. Bettendorf G, Leidenberger F: Amenorrhoea and dysfunctional uterine bleeding in puberty. Clin Endocrinol Metab 1975;4:89.
4. Huffman JW, Dewhurst Sir CJ, Capraro VJ: The gynecology of childhood and adolescence. Philadelphia, WB Saunders, 1981:198–199.
5. Shawker TH, Garra BS, Loriaux DL, et al: Ultrasonography of Turner's syndrome. J Ultrasound Med 1986;5:125.
6. Lippe BM: Primary ovarian failure. In: Kaplan SA, ed. Clinical pediatric and adolescent endocrinology. Philadelphia, WB Saunders, 1982:286–287.
7. Huffman JW, Dewhurst Sir CJ, Capraro VJ: The gynecology of childhood and adolescence. Philadelphia, WB Saunders, 1981:203.
8. Rosenberg HK, Sherman NH, Tarry WF, et al: Mayer-Rokitansky-Kuster-Hauser syndrome: US aid to diagnosis. Radiology 1986;161:815.
9. Kangarloo H, Sarti DA, Sample WF: Ultrasound of the pediatric pelvis. Semin Ultrasound 1980;1:51.
10. Perez CA, Thomas PRM: Radiation therapy: basic concepts and clinical applications. In: Sutow WW, Fernbach DJ, Vietti TJ, eds. Clinical pediatric oncology. St. Louis, C. V. Mosby, 1984, pp. 198–199.
11. Huffman JW, Dewhurst Sir CJ, Capraro VJ: The gynecology of childhood and adolescence. Philadelphia, WB Saunders, 1981:427–428.
12. Pennell RG, Baltarowich OH, Kurtz AB, et al: Complicated first-trimester pregnancies: evaluation with endovaginal US versus transabdominal technique. Radiology 1987;165:79.
13. Goldzieher JW: Polycystic ovarian disease. Fertil Steril 1981;35:371.
14. Huffman JW, Dewhurst Sir CJ, Capraro VJ: The gynecology of childhood and adolescence. Philadelphia, WB Saunders, 1981:439–440.
15. Hann LH, Hall DH, McArdle CR, et al: Polycystic ovarian disease: sonographic spectrum. Radiology 1984;150:531.
16. Yeh H-C, Futterweit W, Thornton JC: Polycystic ovarian disease: US features in 104 patients. Radiology 1987;163:111.
17. Babaknia A, Calfopoulos P, Jones HW Jr: The Stein-Leventhal syndrome and coincidental ovarian tumors. Obstet Gynecol 1976;47:223.
18. Wu A, Siegel MJ: Sonography of pelvic masses in children: diagnostic predictability. AJR 1987;148:1199.

19. Baltarowich OH, Kurtz AB, Pasto ME, et al: The spectrum of sonographic findings in hemorrhagic ovarian cysts. AJR 1987;148:901.
20. Bass IS, Haller JO, Friedman AP, et al: The sonographic appearance of the hemorrhagic ovarian cyst in adolescents. J Ultrasound Med 1984;3:509.
21. Warner MA, Fleischer AC, Edell SL, et al: Uterine adnexal torsion: sonographic findings. Radiology 1985;154:773.
22. Graif M, Shalev J, Strauss S, et al: Torsion of the ovary: sonographic features. AJR 1984;143:1331.
23. Swayne LC, Love MB, Karasick SR: Pelvic inflammatory disease: sonographic-pathologic correlation. Radiology 1984;151:751.
24. Golden N, Cohen H, Gennari G, et al: The use of pelvic ultrasonography in the evaluation of adolescents with pelvic inflammatory disease. Am J Dis Child 1987;141:1235.
25. Lawson TL: Ectopic pregnancy: criteria and accuracy of ultrasonic diagnosis. AJR 1978;131:153.
26. Yoder IC, Pfister RC: Unilateral hematocolpos and ipsilateral renal agenesis: report of two cases and review of the literature. AJR 1976;127:303.
27. Athey PA: Uterus: abnormalities of size, shape, contour, and texture. In: Athey PA, Hadlock FP, ed. Ultrasound in obstetrics and gynecology. St. Louis, CV Mosby, 1985;173–176.

CHAPTER 8

Sexually Transmitted Diseases

Marian C. Craighill, MD, MPh

Sexually active adolescent females represent a high risk group for sexually transmitted diseases (STDs). Adolescents have a well-known tendency to consider themselves invincible, so they do not take appropriate precautions to prevent infections. They also generally have a strong sense of denial, so they do not seek medical attention even when symptoms start to surface. Adolescents are frequently poor compliers with medication and return appointments. Finally, health care providers are not always equipped to address the needs of an adolescent with STDs as patients fall through the cracks between pediatric and adult health care services. Put together, these factors result in adolescents having the highest age-adjusted rates of STDs among sexually active women.[1] These diseases represent significant potential morbidity and even mortality for these young women. Knowledge of the disease patterns in populations can help direct appropriate efforts at screening, counseling, and treatment.

CHLAMYDIA

Chlamydia trachomatis is one of the most common STDs, with an estimated 4.5 million cases per year.[2] It is an obligate intracellular organism, and infection is frequently asymptomatic. Detection in the past has been limited by the cost and relative inavailability of laboratories performing cultures. However, newer fluorescent monoclonal antibody stains and enzyme immunoassay screening tests, although only about 90% sensitive, are less costly and much more available, thus improving overall detection.

Age is a major risk factor for chlamydia with higher rates among teenagers, making it a particularly important organism to screen for in adolescent

Clinical Practice of Gynecology: **3,** 93–102, 1989
© 1989 Elsevier Science Publishing Co., Inc.
655 Avenue of the Americas, New York, NY 10010

ISSN 1043-3198/89/$3.50

populations. Prevalence rates in asymptomatic populations range from 5% to 9% in college health service surveys,[3,4] 26% in inner-city teen clinics,[5] although 12–18% is more typical of rates in teen-family-planning clinics.[6,7] Lower socioeconomic status (SES) is associated consistently with higher prevalence of infection, and race is an important predictor only in these studies when it reflects difference in SES. Among teenagers in an inner-city setting, no difference in prevalence rates was seen when broken into 13–14, 15–16, or 17–18-year-old groups.[5] In addition, prior history of STDs does not increase likelihood of detection. Therefore, current, not past, behavior is what puts a patient at risk, and no immunity is conveyed by prior infection. Two or more partners in the prior 2 months almost doubles the risk of infection, but a new partner in the last 2 months almost triples the likelihood of a positive culture. Barrier methods of birth control are clearly protective with rates of 3.9% versus 11.5% with oral contraceptives and 9.5% with other birth control methods in a clinic where the overall prevalence was 9.3%.[6] Oral contraceptives are only associated with higher rates of chlamydia in women over 20 years old. This has been hypothesized to be due to an increase in cervical ectopy with oral contraceptives that is less apparent in teenagers because of the physiologic ectopy seen in this group. Some authors have postulated this as the reason teens are at greater risk for chlamydia. However, it is unclear whether ectopy itself is a risk factor or whether the more ready accessibility of endocervical cells in this condition enhances detection of the organism. In high-prevalence groups, the presence of this physical finding can bring the detection rate for chlamydia up to 52%.[5] However, the utility of such physical characteristics as ectopy, ready endocervical bleeding, or mucopurulent exudate for making a presumptive diagnosis or for targeting screening tests depends on the population prevalence. Although methodologies and criteria are not uniform between studies, the trend suggests that many more asymptomatic cases will be missed in a high-prevalence population if screening is done selectively than in a low-prevalence group, where such a strategy may be more defendable. However, given the overall cost of long-term morbidity of this disease, routine screening in groups with low-prevalence rates may be cost-effective depending on the screening tool used. Given that primary care practices have reported chlamydia prevalence of 4–9%,[8,9] routine screening among adolescents should be strongly considered.

GONORRHEA

Gonorrhea, unlike chlamydia, is a reportable disease, so national statistics are available at approximately 1 million cases per year, although an estimated 2–9 million cases per year are thought to go unreported. This makes it the most common reportable communicable disease in the United States. Since the 1960s, there has been a dramatic rise in gonorrhea among teenagers, with a peak in 1975 and a relative stabilization of rates since. The increase was the most dramatic in the 10–14-year-old age group. This increase can be attributed to, first, changes in state laws that permitted the treatment of minors for STDs without parental consent leading to better detection and reporting, and, second, to changes in sexual mores resulting in more infection.[10] Two-thirds of all gonorrhea cases are in people between ages 15 and 24 with one-quarter of the cases between the ages of 15 and 19.[11] Rates in female teenagers have consistently exceeded male teen rates since the early 1970s, with a much more marked differential in the 10–14-year-old group.[10] The prevalence of the condition is contributed to by the large number of asymptomatic cases, including 80% of female and 40% of males. The incidence rates (or number of new cases per year) quoted by the Centers for Disease Control (CDC) of approximately 1,400 per 100,000 females age 15–19 per year, or 1 in 61, is somewhat misleading because the appropriate denominator is not all females but rather all sexually active females. When corrected in this fashion, the rate increases from 1,400 to 3,500 cases per 100,000.[1] By way of comparison, the prevalence of positive gonococci (GC) cultures in the above referenced chlamydia studies showed rates from less than 1% to 6%.[6,7] The highest rate among asymptomatic patients was found in inner-city teens with cervical ectopy, who had a rate of 19%.[5]

A seasonal variation in incidence has been recognized since before the era of antibiotics with the highest number of cases in mid- to late summer and a smaller peak a month after Christmas. These patterns are thought to relate to the greater social mobility associated with times when school is not in session. It also reinforces the concept of gonorrhea as a disease of young people.[12]

When adolescents are screened for gonorrhea, it is important to remember that the disease can be transmitted by modes other than sexual intercourse. The gonococcal organism can live in all mucous membranes, including the oral cavity. Surveys of adolescent sexual practices report oral sex in up to two-thirds of teenagers. Therefore, the throat should also be cultured for GC when a sore throat fails to respond to standard treatment in a sexually active adolescent. There are some reports that suggest that gonorrhea can be transmitted by kissing alone.[11]

Penicillin-resistant strains of gonorrhea were first reported in February 1976 and have become the more prevalent type in parts of Asia and Africa. The rates in the United States remain low but continue on an upward trend. This concern emphasizes the need to do sensitivities on all cultures and to always follow up with a test of cure.[12]

PID

The etiologic agent in PID is often unknown, but gonorrhea and chlamydia are certainly the most commonly associated organisms. This serious sequelae is a particularly frequent outcome in young teenagers, developing in one out of every eight sexually active 15-year-olds. This rate falls to one in ten sexually active 16-year-olds, but only one in 80 women over 24.[11] This change in rates of PID with age is much more dramatic than the change in incidence of gonorrhea with age, which suggests some other factor influencing susceptibility. It has been postulated that the physiologic state of the cervix undergoing pubertal maturation at this stage permits much easier access of ascending infection, accounting for the very high rates of pelvic inflammatory disease (PID) in young teenagers.

Estimates of hospitalization rates for PID peaked at 47,000 in 1977 but then came down somewhat to 45,000 per year in the 1980s.[13] These statistics are somewhat obscured by the fact that the diagnosis of PID is not commonly made in a definitive manner. Failure to take a careful and confidential sexual history can lead both to missing the diagnosis as well as treating with antibiotics other conditions, such as functional cysts or early endometriosis. In Scandinavian countries where laparoscopy prior to initiating treatment is a much more common practice, the clinical diagnosis is generally substantiated only 70% of the time.[11] If a laparoscopy is done, it is important to take intraabdominal samples for culture of both GC and chlamydia.

Use of age-specific hospitalization rates for PID can also be somewhat misleading because the criterion for hospitalizing adolescents is often appropriately different from the indications for adults. It is argued that first-episode PID should be treated more aggressively than chronic or recurrent PID. The likelihood of significantly decreasing long-term morbidity, such as infertility or subsequent ectopic pregnancies, is felt to be much better if intravenous antibiotics are used very early in the initial episode, resulting in more hospital admissions for mild disease among adolescents. In addition, poor compliance in teens is also a factor that leads to a greater utilization of hospital-based therapy, thereby skewing comparative statistics. However, given the overall picture of major morbidity from PID with the very significant consequences of infertility, chronic pelvic pain, and ectopic pregnancies, empiric therapy prior to full-blown symptoms is well warranted in adolescents. There should be a low threshold for hospital admission to treat with intravenous (IV) antibiotics early in the course of disease and laparoscopy to confirm the diagnosis if the picture is equivocal. This is true particularly if appendicitis is being considered, because a delay in surgical therapy in this condition can, in fact, increase the chance of a more major infectious process with greater consequent tubal disease.[13]

SYPHILIS

Total syphilis cases have plummeted dramatically since the 1940s, but 1,500–2,000 cases per year are still reported in women 15–19 years old.

Male rates are comparable to female rates in the teen years but then rise sharply after age 20.[14] Seventy percent of men with syphilis have had homosexual contact, which makes this group the largest reservoir of the disease in the United States.[12] A very recent increase in syphilis is thought to be due to interaction with the human immunodeficiency virus (HIV—see below), resulting in a more fulmanant and progressive course to the disease.[1] This trend suggests the need to maintain a close vigilance for this condition.

TRICHOMONAS VAGINALIS

Trichomonas is a sexually transmitted protozoan that is exceedingly common. It is not a reportable disease and has no major morbidity associated with it but does serve as an important marker of sexual activity in the adolescent, and it is often associated with other STDs. The vaginal discharge it may elicit can be the presenting symptom that should elicit culturing for chlamydia and GC. The infection can be dormant for significant periods of time and only be diagnosed incidentally with a Papanicolaou smear. Treatment should include the partner, or recurrence is very likely. Early pregnancy should be excluded prior to treatment with metronidazole, but this recommendation is based entirely on theoretical rather than epidemiologic evidence of problems.[13]

HERPES SIMPLEX VIRUS

Both type I and type II herpes simplex virus (HSV) can cause genital lesions. Type II HSV, however, causes 90% of the genital lesions and recurs much more frequently. Although not reportable as a disease, total new cases are estimated at 300,000–500,000 per year. There are no age-specific data available, but between 1966 and 1982, the number of physician office visits for this condition increased 16 times, suggesting a major increase in the disease.

White patients are much more likely to present with active lesions than other races and frequently may be the first STD they are aware of encountering. This racial difference may be due to differences in utilization of medical services. It may also be due to greater exposure at an earlier age to HSV I or II among nonwhites that conveys some immunity, such that a clinically evident first episode does not develop in the early sexually active years.[12] Serum antibodies are very common with 40–80% positive rates in 14–18-year-olds and often reflect exposure to cold sores rather than genital disease. A culture is really needed to make the diagnosis definitive, although an absent titer acutely followed in 2 weeks by a fourfold rise in the convalescent titers is also definitive, depending on the local laboratory standards. The high prevalence of initial titers, however, makes this a lower-yield workup compared to a properly handled culture swab of a fresh vesicle.[13] Once lesions are at the ulcerative stage, active viral shedding may have ceased. Therefore, the culture swab should be passed over a relatively wide area of involved skin to enhance pickup, with care not to extend to uninvolved areas with possible spread of the virus.

Herpes simplex virus has been linked to cervical dysplasia, although the association is not absolute. It has been hypothesized that HSV acts as an inducer of cell transformation; however, it is clearly not the sole etiologic agent.[12] Nevertheless, young women who have been diagnosed with HSV should have Papanicolaou smears performed regularly and probably at more frequent intervals than noninfected individuals.

HUMAN PAPILLOMAVIRUSES

Human papillomaviruses (HPV) are a group of papova viruses that infect the epithelium primarily. They are categorized by a number representing the order in which they were identified historically. Several are specific to the genital tract, such as HPV types 6, 11, 16, 18, 31, and 33. There is no culture method or serology known; therefore, diagnosis is based on clinical, cytologic, and histologic appearance, or, more recently, on identification of specific viral DNA in tissue. Therefore, any quotation of disease incidence or prevalence will depend on which of these diagnostic criteria are used. However, by available criteria there has been a very marked increase in infection rates in the last several decades. The number of private physician visits for genital warts rose 6.7 times from 1966 to 1984, going from 169,000 to 946,000 visits per year. Among these there was a 4.5-fold increase in first visits for this condition from 53,560 to 224,900 per year, presumably representing new cases. These statistics exclude STD clinics, where a great number of such cases presents, and so grossly underestimate the true totals.[15] In an inner-city teen clinic, there was a 13% prevalence of HPV DNA with the use of southern blot hybridization techniques on cervical scrapings.[16]

While most readily diagnosed, clinically apparent external warts or condyloma acuminata represent only one of many manifestations of HPV infection. In 1976, Meisels[17] pointed out that histologic findings, which have long been considered indicative of early dysplasia, were actually evidence of HPV infection. This caused a large proportion of dysplasias to be reclassified and also directed attention to the association of HPV with cervical and anogenital neoplasia. Cervical cancer had long been associated epidemiologically with sexual activity in patterns that strongly suggested a sexually communicable agent. Up to the point of Meisels' observation, numerous agents had been proposed over time, but none of these had stood up to true scrutiny. Now, HPV genomes have been identified in metastatic cervical cancer cells and are associated with more than 90% of cervical cancers. Recent work using DNA probes has demonstrated that the actual history of a dysplastic lesion is strongly influenced by the specific viral subtype involved. Human papillomavirus 6 or 11 lesions, the typical exophytic warts seen on the vulva and on the cervix, are much less likely to evolve into invasive cancer, although they have the potential for that to occur, while HPV 16, 18, 31, or 33 lesions are much less apparent on the vulva, often appearing only as flat, subclinical lesions. On the cervix, they have a greater propensity to progress, such that a majority of cervical cancers are associated with HPV 16.[18]

Human papillomavirus infection poses a special problem for adolescents because the hormonal changes of puberty induce a normal squamous metaplasia of the transition zone between endo- and exocervix. This environment makes the cervix vulnerable to the initiation of neoplasia when exposed to papilloma virus infection.[16] Other cofactors can also be involved, such as cigarette smoking or concomitant herpes virus infection.[12] Pregnancy, particularly the first pregnancy, also represents a time when HPV infection is more likely to result in dysplasia caused by the high estrogen activity resulting in extensive squamous metaplasia.[16] A history of disequilibrium syndrome (DES) exposure in utero also can be associated with a larger area of squamocolumnar junction, thereby increasing the risk.[19] Host factors clearly play a very large role in the course of a lesion with spontaneous regression seen both in condylomatous lesions as well as dysplasias. Biopsy of a lesion can mobilize a host response that in some cases will totally eliminate the lesion.[20]

Immunosuppression, for whatever reason, is associated with a high rate of malignant transformation, as well as papillomas that are exceedingly hard to eradicate.[21] These malignancies can be anywhere in the anogenital area and can involve more than one viral type.[22]

The clinical implications of these findings are that HPV infection in any part of the genital tract should lead to careful observation for signs of dysplasia or HPV infection. Papanicolaou smears can have a very high false negative rate even in the best of hands and, therefore, should be performed more frequently in adolescents, particularly in the several months after exposure to a new partner or after a pregnancy. A single abnormal Papanicolaou smear, even if it shows only viral effect and no dysplasia per se, should be further investigated with culposcopy.

HUMAN IMMUNODEFICIENCY VIRUS

Human immunodeficiency virus is an STD that causes acquired immunodeficiency disease syndrome (AIDS). On a world wide scale, HIV is most commonly transmitted through vaginal intercourse.[23] The particular circumstances of how the infection was first disseminated in the United States, as well as the 8–10-year lag time generally seen between infection and active disease, means the current bulk of the disease is now in homosexual and bisexual men. Aggressive educational efforts have been successful in curtailing new infections in this group. However, since infection is also blood born, intravenous drug users are currently the group most actively spreading the disease both through contaminated needles and through heterosexual intercourse.[24] This is resulting in a marked increase in the number of HIV-infected women, both as sexual partners of drug users and because one-third of IV drug users are themselves women. Infected women are more likely to be black or Hispanic and to live in the inner city. The highest incidence seen in the United States among women is in the mid-Atlantic states.[25]

The partners of HIV-positive drug users are more likely to be infected than the sexual partners of people who are HIV positive for other reasons, such as from receiving contaminated blood. This suggests that factors other than just frequency of sexual contact affects infectivity.[26] The highest infection rates documented are in men exposed to some African prostitutes with a 5–10% infection rate from a single exposure. Transmission of the virus is more likely if the infected individual is more immunosuppressed. Concurrent STDs, especially ulcerating lesions such as herpes, syphilis, or chancroid, increase the likelihood of transmission. Interestingly, concomitant chlamydia, but not gonorrhea, increases transmission of HIV. To explain this, it has been suggested that chlamydia, but not gonorrhea, may locally mobilize the kind of lymphocyte that HIV infects. Studies in Africa also show greater transmission rates for users of oral contraceptives. It has been postulated that the greater degree of ectropion in oral contraceptive users may be responsible for this finding.[27] This is a particularly disturbing statistic for those attempting to prevent infection among high-risk adolescents.

In New York City, current statistics shows AIDS to be the leading cause of death in young adults. Given the latency period between infection and disease, most of these infections occurred in midadolescence. Ten percent of pediatric AIDS cases are from mothers who are under 21,[1] highlighting the double tragedy of this particular STD with teen pregnancy. From 2% to 3.7% of women attending STD clinics with no known risk factor are HIV positive.[26] Overall, 16% of infected women have no known risk exposure.[25] This emphasizes how difficult it may be for a woman to know her partner's risk factors.

Well-known adolescent behaviors of risk taking, denial, attitudes of invulnerability, and delay in seeking medical services have a very strong potential to spread HIV infection. In doing so, high-risk, inner-city adolescents, through heterosexual transmission, will bridge the infection into the greater community. Only directed, age- and language-appropriate, and aggressive outreach efforts that directly involve the adolescents themselves in creating peer pressure to change behaviors can stem this devastating epidemic.[1]

STDS IN PREPUBERTAL CHILDREN

All of the STDs discussed here should be taken as presumptive evidence of sexual abuse unless maternal transmission during the intrauterine or perinatal period can be documented. Nonsexual human transmission, such as skin-to-skin or skin–mucous–membrane and autoinoculation has been well documented for syphilis and type 1 herpes, but that does not preclude appropriate inquiry.[28] The clinical syndromes are generally similar to what is seen in adolescents, except for gonorrhea, which has a characteristic vulvovaginitis not seen after puberty.[29] Diagnosis of an STD by itself may not prove sexual abuse, but to protect the interests of the child, the health professional must bear the responsibility to demonstrate otherwise.

REFERENCES

1. Hein K, Hurst M: Human immunodeficiency virus infection in adolescence: A rationale for action. Adolesc Pediatr Gynecol 1988;1:73.
2. Washington A, Johnson R, Sanders L, et al: Incidence of Chlamydia trachomatis infections in the United States: Using reported Neisseria gonorrhoeae as a surrogate, in Oriel J, Ridgway G, Schachter J, et al, eds. Chlamydia trachomatis infections: Proceedings of Sixth International Symposium on Human Chlamydia trachomatis Infections. New York: Cambridge University Press, 1986:487–490.
3. McCormack W, Rosner B, McComb D, et al: Infection with Chlamydia trachomatis in female college students. Am J Epidemiol 1985;121:107.
4. Estes K, Robertson S, Sanders J, et al: Incidence of Chlamydia trachomatis in the female student population at the University of Arkansas/Fayetteville. J Arkansas Med Soc 1986;83:217.
5. Chacko M, Lovchik J: Chlamydia trachomatis infection in sexually active adolescents: Prevalence and risk factors. Pediatrics 1984;73:826.
6. Handsfield H, Jasman L, Roberts P, et al: Criteria for selective screening for Chlamydia trachomatis infection in women attending family planning clinics. JAMA 1986;255:1730.
7. Schachter J, Stoner E, Moncada J: Screening for Chlamydial infections in women attending family planning clinics: Evaluation of presumptive indicators for therapy. West J Med 1983;138:375.
8. Berg A, Heidrich F, Fihn S, et al: Establishing the cause of genitourinary symptoms in women in a family practice: Comparison of clinical examination and comprehensive microbiology. JAMA 1984;251:620.
9. Osborne N, Grubin L, Pratson L: Vaginitis in sexually active women: Relationship to nine sexually transmitted organisms. Am J Obstet Gynecol 1982;142:962.
10. Mascola L, Cates W, Reynolds G, et al: Gonorrhea and salpingitis among American teenagers, 1960–1987. MMWR 1983;32:25ss.
11. Phillips S, Spence M: Medical and psychosocial aspects of gonococcal infection in the adolescent patient: Epidemiology, diagnosis, treatment. J Adolesc Health Care 1983;4:128.
12. Perine P, Handsfield H, Holmes K, et al: Epidemiology of the sexually transmitted diseases. Annu Rev Public Health 1985;6:85.
13. Hammill H: Sexually transmitted disease in the female adolescent: Special considerations. Semin Reprod Endocrinol 1988;60:55.
14. Sexually transmitted disease statistics 1984. Atlanta: US Department of Health and Human Services, Public Health Service, Center for Disease Control, Center for Prevention Services, Division of Sexually Transmitted Diseases, 1985.

15. Becker T, Stone T, Alexander E: Genital human papilloma virus infection: a growing concern. Obstet Gynecol Clin North Am 1987;14:389.
16. Garry R, Jones R: Relationship between cervical condylomata, pregnancy and subclinical papilloma virus infection. J Reprod Med 1985;30:393.
17. Meisels A, Fortin R: Condylomatous lesions of the cervix and vagina. I. Cytologic patterns. Acta Cytol (Baltimore) 1976;20:505.
18. Reid R: Human papilloma infection: The key to rational triage of cervical neoplasia. Obstet Gynecol Clin North Am 1987;14:407.
19. Bornstein J, Kaufman R, Adam E, et al: Human papilloma virus associated with vaginal intraepithelial neoplasia in women exposed to diethylstilbesterol in utero. Obstet Gynecol 1987;70:75.
20. Koss L: Dysplasia: A real concept or a misnomer? Obstet Gynecol 1978;51:374.
21. Krebs H, Schneider V, Hurt G, et al: Genital condylomas in immunosuppressed women: A therapeutic challenge. South Med J 1986;79:183.
22. Bergern C, Ferenczy A, Shah K, et al: Multicentric human papilloma virus infection of the female genital tract: Correlations of viral types with mitotic figures culposcopic presentation and location. Obstet Gynecol 1987;69:736.
23. Mann J, Chin J, Pinot P, et al: The international epidemiology of AIDS. Sci Am 1988;259(4):82.
24. Heyward W, Curran J: The epidemiology of AIDS in the U.S. Sci Am 1988;259:72.
25. Quinan M, Hardy A: Epidemiology of AIDS in women in the United States. JAMA 1987;257:2039.
26. Curran J, Jaffe H, Hardy A, et al: Epidemiology of HIV infection and AIDS in the United States. Science 1988;239:610.
27. Piot P, Plummer F, Mhalu F, et al: AIDS: An international perspective. Science 1988;239:573.

CHAPTER 9

Secondary Amenorrhea

Mitchell S. Rein, MD, and Veronica A. Ravnikar, MD

A primary care physician is often notified about the absence of menses or amenorrhea. The evaluation may be initiated by the patient's pediatrician, family practitioner, internist, or gynecologist. There is no universal agreement on the definition of amenorrhea. Traditionally, primary amenorrhea has been defined as the absence of menstruation and secondary sexual characteristics by age 14 or the absence of menstruation by age 16, regardless of secondary sexual characteristics. Secondary amenorrhea has been defined as the absence of menstruation for 3 months or more in women who previously experienced cyclic menstruation. Recently, the distinction between primary and secondary amenorrhea has been deemphasized. This is due largely to the significant overlap of underlying diagnoses. The purpose of this chapter is to provide the clinician with a basic understanding of the clinical entities associated with amenorrhea. A systematic approach to the evaluation of amenorrhea is presented that enables the physician to categorize the causes of amenorrhea into hypothalamic, pituitary, ovarian, or uterine disorders. In the majority of cases, a precise diagnosis can be confirmed, and therapy can be initiated by the primary physician.

HYPOTHALAMIC AMENORRHEA

Exercise-related Amenorrhea

The increasing popularity of regular exercise over the past decade has led to a better understanding of the effects of exercise on the reproductive system. The prevalence of menstrual irregularities in athletic women is reported to be as high as 50%.[1,2] Exercise amenorrhea has been associated

Clinical Practice of Gynecology: **3,** 103–119, 1989
© 1989 Elsevier Science Publishing Co., Inc.
655 Avenue of the Americas, New York, NY 10010
ISSN 1043-3198/89/$3.50

with a variety of sports.[3,4,5] The degree of menstrual dysfunction may be sport specific and associated with the degree of strenuous exercise. The incidence of exercise amenorrhea among long-distance runners is directly correlated with the number of miles run per week and averages between 40–50%, compared to swimmers where the incidence of 12% is independent of training intensity.[4] The influence of age on the development of exercise amenorrhea is highlighted by the observations that strenuous exercise prior to menarche is more likely to produce amenorrhea.[3,5,6] Women who initiate long-distance running prior to the age of 25 are also more likely to develop amenorrhea.[7] The mechanism by which exercise induces amenorrhea appears to be hypothalamic inhibition of GnRH secretion.[8,9] The psychologic and emotional stress associated with exercise may contribute to the hypothalamic inhibition of GnRH secretion (see "Psychogenic Amenorrhea," below). The degree of hypothalamic dysfunction appears to be related to the percentage of body fat. The critical weight hypothesis of Frisch proposes that a minimum ratio of fat to lean mass is normally necessary for menarche (17% fat/body weight) and maintenance of normal menses (22% fat/body weight).[10]

Because of the associated hypoestrogenic hormonal milieu, osteoporosis is a major concern among women with exercise-induced amenorrhea. In contrast, several beneficial effects of exercise have been associated with the prevention of osteoporosis. Modest exercise appears to increase total calcium[11] and lumbar vertebral density.[12] However, bone mineral content has been noted to be reduced among athletes with amenorrhea compared to normal cycling athletes.[13] Bone density of the lumbar spine is lower in amenorrheic runners compared to normal cycling runners and age-matched controls, but higher than in less intense runners with amenorrhea.[14] Although strenuous exercise appears beneficial with regard to osteoporosis and may reduce the impact of amenorrhea on bone loss, patients with exercise-induced amenorrhea remain at high risk for osteoporosis. The management of exercise-related amenorrhea primarily entails recommending modifications of the frequency, duration, and intensity of the particular exercise. Supplemental estrogen and progestin is usually prescribed in the form of an oral contraceptive pill and may prevent accelerated bone loss. Nutritional guidance, including calcium supplementation, may be helpful. When pregnancy is desired, a reduction in exercise and concomitant weight gain should be recommended strongly prior to initiation of ovulation induction.

Weight Loss/Anorexia Nervosa

Weight loss associated with dietary restriction may also result in hypothalamic amenorrhea. As previously mentioned, the critical weight hypothesis of Frisch[10] suggests that a minimum ratio of fat to lean mass (22%) is

Table 9-1. Diagnostic Criteria for Anorexia Nervosa[17]

Age of onset before 25
Weight loss of at least 25% of original body weight
Distorted attitudes including a denial of illness, enjoyment of weight loss, a distorted body
  image and unusual hoarding or handling of food
No known medical illness nor other psychiatric disorder
At least two of the following
  Amenorrhea
  Lanugo
  Bradycardia
  Periods of overactivity
  Episodes of bulimia
  Self-induced emesis

---

required for the maintenance of normal menses. Similar to exercise-related amenorrhea, the mechanism by which food deprivation results in amenorrhea appears to be hypothalamic GnRH dysfunction. Central hypothalamic dysfunction is supported by several findings, including altered regulation of temperature, sleep, thirst, and water conservation[15] and reduced pulsatile LH secretion.[16] Weight-loss-related amenorrhea in its most severe form may be the result of the psychoneuroendocrine disorder anorexia nervosa.

The incidence of eating disorders, including anorexia nervosa and bulimia nervosa, appears to be increasing in Western society. Anorexia nervosa occurs almost exclusively in middle- to upper-class girls under the age of 25. The diagnostic criteria suggested by Feighner[17] is listed in Table 9-1.

Amenorrhea seems to be present in the majority of cases, and some investigators require its presence to establish the diagnosis. The underlying mechanism is central inhibition of GnRH secretion. The amenorrhea may occur before, concurrent with, or after the significant weight loss. In fact, the majority of patients (71%) develop amenorrhea prior to the development of significant weight loss.[18] Even with restoration of normal gonadotropin secretion, approximately 30% of patients remain amenorrheic despite adequate weight gain.[19]

The other clinical features commonly associated with anorexia nervosa are listed in Table 9-2. Many of the signs and symptoms suggest hypothyroidism. Patients with anorexia nervosa usually demonstrate a proportionately greater decrease in triiodothyronine (T_3) compared to thyroxine (T_4). The metabolically inactive reverse $T_3(rT_3)$ is elevated, presumably as a compensatory mechanism to the state of malnutrition.[20] The hypothalamic–pituitary–adrenal axis appears to be activated with hypersecretion of cortisol[21] but also suppression of adrenal androgen secretion.[22] Approximately 50% of patients have partial diabetes insipidus.[23] Hypercarotenemia, a yellowish discoloration of the skin usually seen on the palms, may be used in establishing the diagnosis, since serum carotene levels tend to be decreased in other forms of malnutrition.[24]

Table 9-2. Clinical Features of Anorexia Nervosa

Symptoms	Signs	Laboratory Findings
Constipation	Dry skin	Decreased thyroid function
Cold intolerance	Hypotension	Increased cortisol
Lethargy	Hypothermia	Increased growth hormone
	Bradycardia	Decreased gonadotropins
	Edema	Increased BUN
	Hypercarotenemic	

There is no specific recommended therapy for anorexia nervosa. Early recognition is important so that appropriate psychotherapy can be instituted before the development of severe life-threatening weight loss. Various therapeutic interventions have been advocated with favorable results, including psychoanalysis, family therapy, force feeding, and behavior modification.[25] The usefulness of neuropharmacologic agents remains to be proven; preliminary studies with antidepressants and cyproheptadine have yielded equivocal results. Similar to exercise-related amenorrhea, patients with anorexia nervosa may benefit from estrogen replacement therapy for the prevention of osteoporosis and should be followed with serial bone densitometry to assess the efficacy of estrogen therapy.

Anosmia and Amenorrhea

A rare clinical syndrome of hypogonadotropic hypogonadism similar to Kalmann's syndrome has been reported in females.[26] Although heterogeneous, the syndrome is characterized by amenorrhea, low gonadotropins, anosmia, normal karyotype, and infantile sexual development. Autopsy studies have revealed that the isolated gonadotropin deficiency is associated with partial or complete agenesis of the olfactory lobes.[27] The underlying pathophysiology involves abnormal GnRH production and/or responsiveness.[28] Patients desiring pregnancy can be treated with exogenous gonadotropins. Similar to other forms of hypothalamic amenorrhea, estrogen replacement therapy is recommended to prevent accelerated bone loss.

Postpill Amenorrhea

The incidence of amenorrhea after discontinuation of oral contraceptive pills (OCPs) has been reported to be 2.2 per 1,000 women.[29] However, multiple attempts to demonstrate a cause-and-effect relationship have been unsuccessful.[30,31] An increased incidence among women with previously irregular menstrual cycles seems to suggest an abnormality of the hypothalamic–pituitary–ovarian axis prior to the initiation of OCPs. Therefore, patients with greater than 6 months of postpill amenorrhea require a complete evaluation.

Psychogenic Amenorrhea

In the absence of an organic disease, anatomic defect, and/or specific cause, amenorrhea may develop as a result of psychogenic stress. Psychogenic amenorrhea appears to be more common in unmarried, career-oriented women.[32] Similar to other forms of hypothalamic amenorrhea, patients demonstrate low levels of gonadotropins as a result of impaired GnRH secretion. Management should be directed at identifying and subsequently improving the underlying stress and/or coping mechanisms. Patients should be reassured of the benign nature of psychogenic amenorrhea, particularly regarding future fertility. If amenorrhea persists despite psychologic guidance, estrogen-progestin replacement should be initiated. If pregnancy is desired, ovulation induction may be required.

PITUITARY CAUSES OF AMENORRHEA

Hyperprolactinemia

The association of amenorrhea and high prolactin is well documented.[33] The primary mechanism appears to be hypoestrogenism secondary to inhibition of pulsatile GnRH secretion.[34] Elevated prolactin may also cause direct inhibition of steroidogenesis at the level of the ovary.[35] Patients with hyperprolactinemia and amenorrhea are at risk for the development of osteoporosis.[36] Treatment of hyperprolactinemia in amenorrheic women is associated with resumption of menses and prevention of bone loss.[37] A number of clinical conditions may cause elevated circulating prolactin. These include various medications, chest wall trauma, chronic renal insufficiency, hypothyroidism, empty sella syndrome, pituitary stalk transection, pituitary tumors, and, rarely, nonpituitary tumors. Medications that commonly cause hyperprolactinemia include phenothiazines, tricyclic antidepressants, and estrogen-containing medications, including oral contraceptive agents, butyrophenones, metoclopramide, reserpine, amphetamines, and aldomet. Transient elevations of prolactin have been associated with beer and protein ingestion, herpes zoster, nipple stimulation, stress, sexual intercourse, and hypoglycemia.

Pituitary Tumors

Pituitary tumors are classified as microadenomas (<1 cm) or macroadenomas (>1 cm). Although classically grouped according to their staining characteristics, pituitary tumors are best categorized according to their function. Refinements of computed tomography (CT) have increased the sensitivity of detecting small pituitary tumors. Although CT remains the method of choice for diagnosing pituitary tumors, magnetic resonance imaging (MRI) may replace CT, since it offers excellent resolution without the exposure of ionizing radiation. Even though pituitary adenomas tend to be associated with high levels of prolactin, they may be associated with any degree of hyperprolactinemia. Therefore, we recommend radiographic evaluation with either CT or MRI for *all* patients with persistent hyperprolactinemia regardless of the absolute level.

Prolactin-secreting adenomas are the most common pituitary tumor. They are usually found in the lateral aspects of the pituitary. Although the natural history of prolactinomas is not well defined, tumors are generally slow-growing. Although galactorrhea and amenorrhea are common, not all women with hyperprolactinemia have these symptoms. Less common clinical features include headache, visual disturbances, and, rarely, signs of hyperthyroidism, acromegaly, and hypercortisolism secondary to concomitant thyroid-stimulating hormone (TSH), growth hormone (GH), and corticotropin (ACTH) overproduction. Pregnancy appears to increase the risk of tumor growth, because of the stimulatory effects of estrogen on lactotrophs. Approximately 5–10% of women with microadenomas[38] and 30–40% of women with macroadenomas[39,40] will develop signs and symptoms suggestive of tumor enlargement during pregnancy. Baseline visual field studies should be obtained in any patient with a macroadenoma or in any pregnant patient with a microadenoma.

There is no universal agreement regarding the optimal management of prolactin-secreting pituitary adenomas. However, at the present time, the majority of patients can be treated safely and successfully with medical therapy and avoid the potential morbidity and significant recurrence rate associated with surgical exploration. The dopamine agonist bromocriptine (Parlodel) has been proven efficacious for the treatment of microadenomas[41] and macroadenomas.[42] Patients should *gradually* increase their dose to 2.5 mg twice a day. In the majority of patients, prolactin normalizes, menses resume and galactorrhea improves. Rarely, increasing the dose to 2.5 mg three times a day is required to suppress serum prolactin. Common side effects include nausea, headache, orthostatic hypotension, and nasal congestion.

Transsphenoidal surgical resection is an acceptable alternative therapy, particularly in patients with macroadenomas who are not interested in indefinite bromocriptine therapy. Patients with macroadenomas may also consider primary surgical therapy prior to attempting pregnancy because of the increased risk of tumor extension. Tumor size, tumor extension, significant hyperprolactinemia, and the expertise of the neurosurgeon are important factors that affect the surgical prognosis. Tumors less than 2 cm in diameter and a serum prolactin less than 200 ng/mL are associated with a favorable prognosis.[43] Since preoperative bromocriptine therapy appears to decrease tumor size, it may facilitate surgical exploration and reduce postoperative morbidity. Complete resolution of hyperprolactinemia with resumption of menses will occur in 40% of patients with macroadenomas and 70–80% of patients with microadenomas.[44,45] However, evidence of recurrent tumor growth based on recurrent hyperprolactinemia appears high.[46] Complications of surgery include panhypopituitarism, meningitis, diabetes insipidus, and persistent and recurrent tumor. Because it is less effective than medical or surgical therapy, radiation therapy is rarely recommended as a primary therapy. Cobalt beam or proton beam irradiation may be useful for the treatment of unresectable or partially resectable tumors. Response is very slow, and prolactin levels may take years to fall. Complications are rare, however, and panhypopituitarism of variable degrees may present many years after treatment. Since most tumors are slow-growing, and spontaneous regression may occur, expectant management of microadenomas appears acceptable. Patients should be followed with serial prolactin levels and regular CT or MRI examinations to exclude the possibility of progressive tumor growth. In patients with persistent amenorrhea, estrogen replacement therapy to prevent accelerated bone loss is an acceptable alternative to bromocriptine therapy. Although there is no evidence that OCP use causes pituitary adenomas,[47] theoretic concern over exacerbating growth of a preexisting adenoma remains.

Growth hormone and ACTH-secreting pituitary adenomas have also been associated with hyperprolactinemia and amenorrhea. These pituitary tumors result in the clinical appearance of acromegaly and Cushings Disease, respectively. Less common pituitary tumors include TSH, luteinizing hormone (LH), follicle-stimulating hormone (FSH), and β-endorphin-secreting pituitary adenomas.

Empty Sella Syndrome

Empty sella syndrome is an incompleteness of the sellar diaphragm resulting in the extension of the subarachnoid space into the pituitary fossa. It may be congenital or secondary to surgery or irradiation. The pituitary gland tends to be flattened or displaced upwards. Symptoms may include cerebrospinal fluid (CSF) rhinorrhea, headaches, amenorrhea, and galactorrhea.[48] Patients tend to be middle-aged and obese.[49] The condition is benign, and no particular therapy is required. In patients with elevated prolactins, regular radiographic surveillance is recommended to exclude the possibility of a concomitant tumor. If amenorrhea is present, estrogen replacement therapy is recommended to prevent osteoporosis.

Hypopituitarism

Primary hypopituitarism may result from surgical or radiologic ablation, large pituitary tumors, infarction, or infiltrating and granulomatous lesions. Pituitary infarction may be spontaneous but more commonly is associated with postpartum hemorrhage (Sheehan's syndrome) or pituitary tumors (pituitary apoplexy). Large pituitary tumors are usually nonfunctional. Although generally benign, hypothalamic-pituitary tumors may be life-threatening and should always be considered in the evaluation of amenorrhea. The growth of a benign tumor may cause headache, visual impairment, and varying degrees of hypopituitarism. The most common visual field defect is bitemporal hemianopsia secondary to compression of the optic chiasm. Craniopharyngiomas, arising from remnants of Rathke's pouch, are the most common nonpituitary tumor associated with hyperprolactinemia and are a common cause of hypothalamic hypopituitarism. Craniopharyngiomas occur most frequently in the second decade[50] and may present with headache, visual disturbances, and/or amenorrhea. Other hypothalamic tumors include germinoma (ectopic pinealoma), glioma, teratoma, and endodermal sinus tumor (yolk-sac carcinoma). Infiltrating and granulomatous lesions resulting in hypopituitarism include Hand–Schüller–Christian disease (histiocytosis X), tuberculosis, toxoplasmosis, and sarcoidosis. Finally, head trauma, usually as a result of a motor vehicle accident, can cause hypopituitarism from transection of the pituitary stalk.

OVARIAN CAUSES OF AMENORRHEA

Premature Ovarian Failure

Premature ovarian failure (POF) is defined as failure of ovarian estrogen production in the setting of hypergonadotropism before the age of 35. Although most cases are idiopathic, the etiology of POF appears to be multifactorial. Recent evidence supports the hypothesis that a specific genetic defect may cause POF.[51] Premature ovarian failure may be the result of a reduced number of primordial follicles or an increased rate of atresia. Infectious and iatrogenic destruction of primordial follicles may occur as a result of mumps oophoritis, irradiation, or chemotherapy. Documentation of antiovarian antibodies and the association of POF with other immunologic endocrine disorders supports the hypothesis that POF may be an autoimmune disease.[52] An increased incidence of POF has also been associated with abnormal galactose metabolism.[53]

The clinical presentation of POF is quite variable. Patients may present at varying ages with primary or secondary amenorrhea. Symptoms suggestive of menopause include hot flashes, vaginal dryness, and sleep and mood disturbances. Ovarian failure may be temporary with spontaneous return of menstrual function. Associated autoimmune disorders include Addison's disease, thyroiditis, hypoparathyroidism, diabetes, pernicious anemia, myasthenia gravis, and vitiligo. Because of the associated polyendocrine autoimmune syndromes, patients should be screened for diabetes, anemia, and thyroid, adrenal and parathyroid insufficiency.

The diagnosis is confirmed by elevated gonadotropins, particularly FSH. Although postmenopausal levels of gonadotropins are very reliable, there are several *rare* clinical entities in which high gonadotropins are associated with ovaries that contain follicles. The resistant or insensitive ovary syndrome represents an absence of gonadotropin receptors on the follicles. Neoplastic tumors can produce gonadotropins. An isolated LH or FSH deficiency will result in elevation of the other gonadotropin in association with amenorrhea. A selective elevation of FSH has been attributed to inadequate production of inhibin. The 17 hydroxylase enzyme deficiency results in a decreased production of adrenal and gonadal steroids with associated absent secondary sexual development, primary amenorrhea, hypertension, and elevated gonadotropins.

All patients with POF under the age of 30 should have a chromosomal analysis to identify gonadal dysgenesis and possible mosaicism. Although Turner's syndrome (XO) is generally associated with primary amenorrhea, Turner's mosaicism (XX/XO) may be associated with varying degrees of female development and POF. Unlike patients with Turner's syndrome, these patients may appear normal. The major reason for obtaining a karyotype is to identify any patients with a Y chromosome. A palpable uterus, distinguishes XY gonadal dysgenesis (Swyer's syndrome) from testicular feminization (TF). Except for patients with a complete form of TF, all patients with a Y chromosome, including mosaics, should undergo gonadectomy before puberty to avoid gonadal neoplasia and virilization. If one is over the age of 30, the possibility of a gonadal tumor is extremely rare, and, therefore, genetic evaluation is not necessary.

Management of patients with POF should concentrate on estrogen/progestin replacement for the prevention of osteoporosis, and possibly cardiovascular disease. Serial bone densitometry should be considered, particularly in patients at risk for the development of osteoporosis. Ovulation can rarely be induced. However, the possibility of spontaneous resumption of ovarian function makes it difficult to tell most patients they are permanently sterile.

Polycystic Ovary Syndrome (PCOS)

It has become increasingly clear that PCOS is a heterogenous disease. Although the exact pathophysiology remains controversial, recent reviews have suggested a multifactorial etiology.[54] At least five major systems may contribute to the development of PCOS: 1) hypothalamus/pituitary, 2) ovary, 3) skin, 4) adrenal, and/or 5) pancreas. The symptoms associated with PCOS include amenorrhea, hirsutism, infertility, dysfunctional uterine bleeding, obesity, and dysmenorrhea. In the past, the diagnosis was based on the anatomic findings of polycystic or sclerocystic ovaries (Stein–Leventhal syndrome). However, women with classic symptoms and hormonal parameters suggestive of PCOS may have normal-appearing ovaries. Conversely, polycystic ovaries may be observed in women with specific causes of hyperandrogenism, including Cushing's syndrome, congenital adrenal hyperplasia, ovarian and adrenal tumors, hyperprolactinemia, hypothyroidism, and acromegaly. As a result, there is no universal agreement regarding the diagnostic criteria for PCOS. More recently, there has been an attempt to subclassify the heterogenous PCOS into distinct disease subgroups based on specific biochemical abnormalities. The characteristic biochemical abnormalities include ovarian hyperandrogenism, inappropriate gonadotropin secretion, peripheral hyperestrogenism, and hyperinsulinemia.

The inappropriate gonadotropin secretion involves an elevated level of LH and a normal or low level of FSH. Some authors have advocated an elevated LH:FSH ratio of greater than 3 as diagnostic of PCOS.[55] However, some patients with PCOS may have normal gonadotropins. The mechanisms that are responsible for inappropriate gonadotropin secretion remain to be fully elucidated. Centrally, a relative deficiency of dopamine[56] and a relative excess of norepinephrine[57] may contribute to the elevated secretion of LH. Peripherally, relatively constant levels of estrogen (derived from extraglandular conversion of androstenedione) appear to contribute to the increased sensitivity of the pituitary to GnRH stimulation of LH release and decreased pituitary secretion of FSH.[58] Finally, an increased secretion of inhibin may contribute to the selective inhibition of FSH secretion.[59]

The association of hyperinsulinemia with PCOS has been manifested clinically by acanthosis nigricans and termed the HAIR-AN syndrome (hyperandrogenism, insulin resistance, acanthosis nigricans).[60] The severity of the insulin resistance is strongly correlated with the degree of hyperinsulinemia, which in turn is highly correlated with the severity of the hyperandrogenism. Although the exact mechanisms remain to be fully elucidated in vivo[61] and in vitro,[62,63] evidence suggests that the hyperinsulinemic state causes the hyperandrogenism and not vice versa. This is further supported by the observation that the insulin resistance and acanthosis nigricans is not affected by lowering ovarian androgen production.[54] Among women with significant ovarian hyperandrogenism (serum testosterone >1 ng/mL), approximately 50% will demonstrate insulin resistance[61] while only 5% have acanthosis nigricans.[64]

The management of PCOS is directed according to the patients' specific complaints. In patients with amenorrhea, hirsutism, or dysfunctional uterine bleeding, treatment with oral contraceptive pills (OCPs) may restore normal menses and improve ovarian hyperandrogenism. Endometrial sampling should be considered prior to ovulation induction and occasionally prior to the initiation of OCPs, since patients are at risk for endometrial hyperplasia because of the hyperestrogenic anovulatory state. Ovulation induction with clomiphene citrate is often successful in patients with associated infertility.

UTERINE CAUSES OF AMENORRHEA

Congenital Malformations

Müllerian agenesis (Mayer–Rokitansky–Kuster–Hauser syndrome) and a number of other müllerian anomalies, including testicular feminization, are a major cause of primary amenorrhea. These clinical entities are further discussed in Chapter 13.

Asherman's Syndrome

Asherman's syndrome may cause secondary amenorrhea as a result of uterine and/or cervical synechia. The amenorrhea may be due to an inadequate uterine cavity, the obstruction of menstrual flow and/or the inability of the endometrium to respond to hormonal stimuli. A strict definition or diagnostic criteria are lacking for Asherman's syndrome. The adhesions may be variable in location with partial or complete obliteration of the uterine cavity and/or cervical canal. Patients may present with symptoms other than amenorrhea, including cyclic painful hypomenorrhea, menstrual irregularities, infertility, and habitual abortion. Asherman's syndrome is almost always associated with trauma and/or infection.

The most common etiology is an aggressive, postpartum, or postabortal dilatation and curettage. Cases have been reported following cesarean section, myomectomy, and metroplasty. Although associated endometritis is quite common, an isolated infectious etiology in the absence of trauma is rare. Cases have been reported following polymicrobial, tuberculosis, schistosomiasis, and IUD-related endomyometritis. The diagnosis may be strongly suspected by the patient's history. However, it is best confirmed by hysteroscopy. The correlation between hysterosalpingograms and hysteroscopic findings appear poor.[65] In patients with secondary amenorrhea, the absence of withdrawal bleeding, after a provera challenge, suggests severe hypoestrogenism and/or Asherman's syndrome. Patients with uterine causes of amenorrhea should have normal endocrine function with evidence of ovulation.

The optimal treatment for Asherman's syndrome remains to be defined. The goals of therapy are removal of the adhesions, and maintenance of the uterine cavity. Hysteroscopic removal of adhesions may be more complete than the "blind" D&C. Insertion of a Foley catheter at the time of adhesiolysis for an appropriate period of time may help maintain the integrity of the uterine cavity and may be more effective than an intrauterine device (IUD). Broad spectrum antibiotic therapy is strongly recommended pre- and postoperatively. Finally, hormonal therapy with high doses of estrogen and provera to stimulate regeneration and separation of the endometrium is recommended though the optimal dosage and duration of therapy has not been established.

THE EVALUATION OF AMENORRHEA

The evaluation of amenorrhea is actually quite simple. A systematic approach is presented that enables the clinician to categorize the causes of amenorrhea into hypothalamic, pituitary, ovarian or uterine disorders (see Figure 9-1). Most of the time, a specific etiology can be confirmed. The workup should begin with a careful history and physical exam. Patients should be questioned about sexual activity, symptoms of pregnancy, nutritional status, stress, galactorrhea, headaches, visual disturbances, hot flashes, hirsutism, medications, medical, surgical, and family history. It is extremely important to rule out pregnancy as a possible cause of amenorrhea prior to pursuing an extensive evaluation. The physical exam should focus on signs of pregnancy, body habitus, secondary sexual development, internal and external genitalia, galactorrhea, hirsutism, and thyromegaly. Initial laboratory studies should include a beta subunit, prolactin, thyroid function tests, FSH, and total testosterone.

After these tests, a progesterone challenge test should be performed. The purpose of the progesterone challenge test is to assess the patency of the uterine cervical/vaginal outflow tract and to estimate the level of endogenous estrogen. Patients can be treated with a single intramuscular injection of 200 mg of progesterone in oil or medroxyprogesterone acetate (Provera) 10 mg orally for 5 days. Bleeding of any amount is considered positive and will usually occur within 2–7 days. A positive test confirms the presence of adequate endogenous estrogen and a patent outflow tract, and suggests anovulation.

Patients with a negative progesterone challenge test should be challenged with a combination of estrogen and progestin (OCPs) to distinguish outflow tract obstruction from hypoestrogenism. All patients with evidence of hypoestrogenism (negative progesterone; positive estrogen/progestin challenge), regardless of the underlying etiology, should be recommended estrogen replacement therapy to prevent accelerated bone loss. The absence of withdrawal bleeding after combination therapy is strongly suggestive of a uterine cause of amenorrhea. However, patients with mild to moderate Asherman's syndrome may bleed following estrogen and progestin therapy. Therefore, if the patient's history is suggestive of Asherman's syndrome, hysteroscopic evaluation should be considered. Patients with severe hypoestrogenism as documented by a negative progesterone challenge and positive estrogen/progestin challenge test should have a lateral-coned-down view of the sella turcica and/or a head CT scan to exclude the small possibility of hypothalamic-pituitary tumor.

Elevated prolactin is often suggestive of a pituitary disorder. The controversies regarding the evaluation and treatment of an elevated prolactin have been previously discussed. A radiographic evaluation with CT or MRI is required to rule out a hypothalamic-pituitary tumor. In the absence of a tumor, the other causes of hyperprolactinemia should be considered.

Secondary Amenorrhea
Obtain βhCG
Positive Pregnancy
Negative
Obtain Height/Weight
Prolactin (PRL)
FSH
Testosterone (Testo)
Dehydroepiandrosterone (DS) (if indicated)
17–OH Progesterone (if indicated)
Thyroid Function Tests
Progesterone Withdrawal (PW) (after blood tests)
Abnormal Height/Weight
↑ PRL
↑ FSH
↑ Testosterone
PW (+) (Anovulation)
PW (−)
Obese
Excessively Thin
CT or MRI of the Hypothalamus/ Pituitary
Premature Ovarian Failure (consider Chromosomes) (consider Auto-immune Disorders)
↑ LH/FSH (PCOS)
Testo (>2ng/ml) DS (>7000ng/ml)
(+) Estrogen/Progestin (nl PRL, FSH, Testo)
(−) Estrogen/Progestin
rule out:
PCOS
Cushings Disease
Exercise Anorexia Nervosa
(+)
(−)
Hypothalamic Pituitary Tumor
rule out:
Hypothyroidism
Drugs
Renal Failure
Chest Wall Trauma
Empty Sella Syndrome
rule out: (Androgen Producing Tumors) (Ovarian Hyper-thecosis)
rule out:
Hypoth-Pit Tumor Asherman's Syndrome
Cong Malformations Asherman's Syndrome
Hypothalamic Amenorrhea

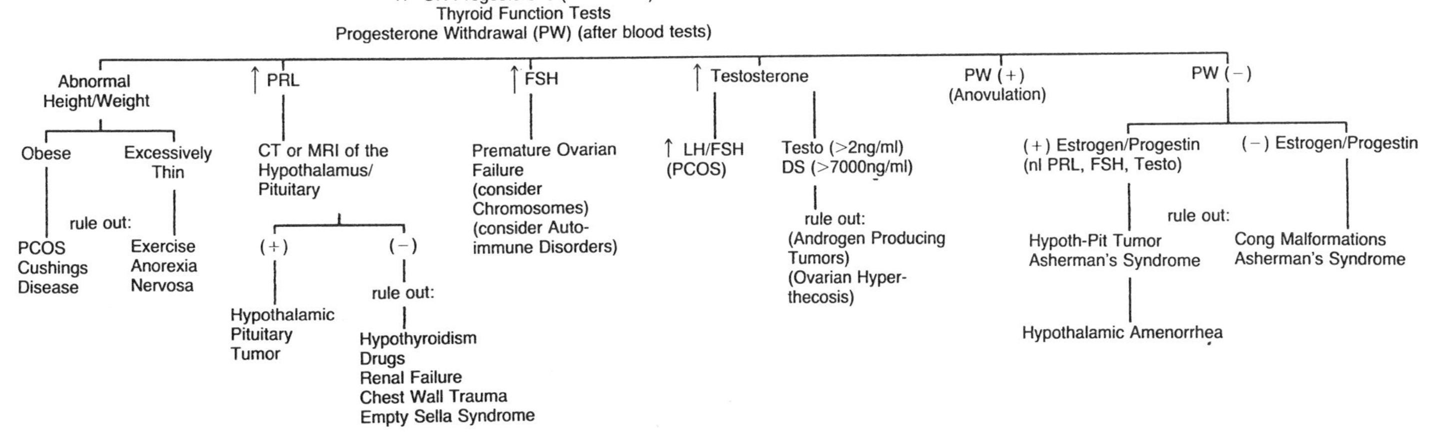

FIGURE 9-1

An elevated FSH is strongly suggestive of POF. Rare causes of elevated gonadotropins have been previously discussed; however, routine laparoscopic or open ovarian biopsy to determine the patient's follicular status is not recommended. Patients under the age of 30 are recommended a chromosomal analysis to rule out the possibility of a Y chromosome and/or mosaicism.

Patients with elevated testosterone most often have some form of PCOS. This may be confirmed by a LH:FSH ratio of greater than 3. Patients with Cushing's disease may clinically appear similar to patients with PCOS, and can be distinguished from PCOS with a dexamethasone suppression test. In patients with signs of hirsutism and/or virilization, an elevated 17-hydroxyprogesterone level suggests adrenal hyperplasia. The diagnosis of adrenal hyperplasia is best confirmed with an ACTH stimulation test. Signs of virilization may also be seen with ovarian stromal hyperthecosis and androgen-producing tumors. Patients with hirsutism should also have a dehydroepiandosterone sulfate level to exclude the rare possibility of an adrenal tumor. Patients with significant ovarian hyperandrogenism may also have acanthosis nigricans and insulin resistance.

Hypothalamic amenorrhea is a diagnosis of exclusion. Although stress, weight loss, and exercise are commonly associated, there may be no obvious underlying cause. Gonadotropins are normal or low, and the progestin challenge is negative.

SUMMARY

Irregular menstrual cycles and/or subsequent amenorrhea continues to be a common problem among the pediatric patient population. The primary care physician should be familiar with the differential diagnosis and the initial evaluation. In the majority of cases, a specific etiology can be confirmed. The causes of amenorrhea and our approach to the evaluation of amenorrhea has been presented. It is particularly important to identify patients with hypothalamic-pituitary tumors and patients at risk for the development of osteoporosis. Therapy should be individualized according to the patient's underlying disorder and her immediate goals, ie, resumption of menses versus pregnancy.

REFERENCES

1. Garner PR: The effect of body weight on menstrual function. Curr Prob/Obstet Gynecol 1984;4:1.
2. Webb JL, Millan DL, Stolz CJ: Gynecological survey of American female athletes competing at the Montreal Olympic Games. J Sports Med Phys Fitness 1979;19:405.
3. Frisch RE, Gotz-Welbergen AV, McArthur JW, et al: Delayed menarche and amenorrhea of college athletes in relation to age of onset of training. JAMA 1981;246:1559.

4. Sanborn CF, Martin BJ, Wagner WW: Is athletic amenorrhea specific to runners? Am J Obstet Gynecol 1982;143:859.

5. Frisch RE, Wyshak G, Vincent LE: Delayed menarche and amenorrhea in ballet dancers. N Engl J Med 1980;303:17.

6. Warren MP: The effects of exercise on pubertal progression and reproductive function in girls. J Clin Endocrinol Metab 1980;51:1150.

7. Speroff L: The effect of exercise on the menstrual cycle. Postgrad Obstet Gynecol 1984;4:1.

8. Reame NE, Sander SE, Case GD, et al: Pulsatile gonadotropin secretion in women with hypothalamic amenorrhea: Evidence that reduced frequency of gonadotropin-releasing hormone secretion is the mechanism of persistent anovulation. J Clin Endocrinol Metab 1985;61:851.

9. Comming DC, Vickovie MM, Wall SR, et al: Defects in pulsatile LH release in normally menstruating runners. J Clin Endocrinol Metab 60;810:1985.

10. Frisch RE, McArthur JW: Menstrual cycles. Fatness as a determinant of minimum weight for height necessary for their maintenance or onset. Science 1974;185:949.

11. Aloia JF, Cohn M, Osinni JA, et al: Prevention of involutional bone loss by exercise. Ann Intern Med 1978;89:356.

12. Krolner B, Toft B, Nielson SP, et al: Physical exercise as prophylaxis against involutional vertebral bone loss: A controlled trial. Clin Sci 1983;64:541.

13. Drinkwater BL, Nilson K, Chestnut CH, et al: Bone mineral content of amenorrheic and eumenorrheic athletes. N Engl J Med 1984;311:277.

14. Marcus RC, Cann P, Maduig J, et al: Menstrual function and bone mass in elite women distance runners. Ann Intern Med 1985;102:158.

15. Vigersky RA, Loriaux DL: Anorexia Nervosa. New York: Raven Press, 1977:109.

16. Kapen SE, Sternthal. Braverman. Case report. A pubertal 2-hour luteinizing hormone (LH) secretory pattern following weight loss in the absence of anorexia nervosa. Psychosom Med 1981;43:177.

17. Feighner JP, Robins E, Guze SB, et al: Diagnostic criteria for use in psychiatric research. Arch Gen Psychiatry 1972;26:57–63.

18. Fries H: Studies on secondary amenorrhea, anorectic behavior, and body-image perception: Importance for the early recognition of anorexia nervosa. In: Vigersky RA, ed. Anorexia nervosa. New York: Raven Press, 1977:163–76.

19. Warren MP, VandeWiele RL: Clinical and metabolic features of anorexia nervosa. Am J Obstet Gynecol 1973;117:435.

20. Bray GA, Fisher DA, Chopra J: Relation of thyroid hormones to body weight. Lancet 1976; i:1206.

21. Doerr P, Fichter M, Pirke KM, et al: Relationship between weight gain and hypothalamic pituitary adrenal function in patients with anorexia nervosa. J Steroid Biochem 1980;13:529.

22. Zumoff B, Walsh BT, Katz JL, et al: Subnormal plasma dehydroisoandrosterone to cortisol ratio in anorexia nervosa: A second hormonal parameter of ontogenic regression. J Clin Endocrinol Metab 1983;56:668.

23. Meckelbury RS, Loriaux DL, Thompson RM, et al: Hypothalamic dysfunction in patients with anorexia nervosa. Medicine 1974;53:147.

24. Schwabe AD, Pope MA: The role of the gastrointestinal tract in carotene and vitamin A metabolism. Arq Gastroenterol 1975;12:269–272.

25. Lucas AR, Duncan JA, Piens V: The treatment of anorexia nervosa. Am J Psychiatry 1976;133:1034.

26. Tagate G, Fialkou PJ, Smith D, et al: Hypogonadotropic hypogonadism associated with anosmia in the female. N Engl J Med 1970;282:1326.

27. DeMorsier G: Etudes sur les dysrapmies cranioencepaliques. Schweiz Arch Neurol Neurochir Psychiatr 1954;74:309.

28. Crowley WF, Filcori M, Spratt D, et al: The physiology of gonadotropin releasing hormone (GnRH) secretion in men and women. Recent Prog Horm Res 1985;41:473.

29. Golditch LM: Postcontraceptive amenorrhea. Obstet Gynecol 1972;39:903.

30. Jacobs MS, Knuth VA, Hull MGR, et al: Postpill amenorrhea—cause or coincidence? Br Med J 1977;2:940.

31. Tolis G: Prolonged amenorrhea and oral contraceptives. Fertil Steril 1979;32:265.

32. Fries M, Nillius SJ, Petterson F: Epidemiology of secondary amenorrhea. II. A retrospective evaluation of etiology with special regard to psychogenic factors and weight loss. Am J Obstet Gynecol 1974;118:473.

33. Jacobs HS: Prolactin and amenorrhea. N Engl J Med 1976;295:954.

34. Monroe SE, Levine L, Chany RJ, et al: Prolactin-secreting pituitary adenomas. V. Increased gonadotropin responsivity in hyperprolactinemic women with pituitary adenomas. J Clin Endocrinol Metab 1981;52:1171.

35. McNatty KP, Sawers RS, McNeilly AS: A possible role for prolactin in control of steroid secretion by the human graafian follicle. Nature 1973;250:653.

36. Klibanski A, Neer RM, Beitins IZ, et al: Decreased bone density in hyperprolactinemic women. N Engl J Med 1980;303:1511.

37. Klibanski A, Greenspan SL: Increase in bone mass after treatment of hyperprolactinemic amenorrhea. N Engl J Med 1980;315:542.

38. Jewelewicz R, Vande Wiele RL: Clinical course and outcome of pregnancy in twenty-five patients with pituitary microadenomas. Am J Obstet Gynecol 1980;136:339.

39. Magyar DM, Marshall JR: Pituitary tumors and pregnancy. Am J Obstet Gynecol 1978;132:739.

40. Gemzell C, Wang CF: Outcome of pregnancy in women with pituitary adenoma. Fertil Steril 1979;31:363.

41. Archer DF, Laftanzi DR, Moore EE, et al: Bromocriptine treatment of women with suspected pituitary prolactin-secreting microadenoma. Am J Obstet Gynecol 1982;143:620.

42. Hancock KW, Scott JS, Lamb JT, et al: Conservative management of pituitary prolactinomas. Evidence for bromocriptine induced regression. Br J Obstet Gynaecol 1980;87:523.

43. Keye WR Jr, Chang RJ, Monroe SE, et al: Prolactin-secreting pituitary adenomas in women. II. Menstrual function, pituitary reserves and prolactin production following microsurgical removal. Am J Obstet Gynecol 1979;134:360.

44. Woosley RE, King JS, Talbert L: Prolactin-secreting pituitary adenomas: Neurosurgical management of 37 patients. Fertil Steril 1982;37:54.

45. Post KD, Biller BJ, Adelman, et al: Selective transsphenoidal adenomectomy in women with galactorrhea, amenorrhea. JAMA 1979;242:158.

46. Serri O, Rasio E, Beaureyard M, et al: Recurrence of hyperprolactinemia after selective transsphenoidal adenomectomy in women with prolactinoma. N Engl J Med 1983;309:280.

47. Pituitary adenoma study group. Pituitary adenomas and oral contraceptives. A multicenter case-control study. Fertil Steril 1983;39:753.

48. Neelon FA, Goree JA, Lebovitz ME: The primary empty sella. Clinical and radiographic characteristics and endocrine function. Medicine 1973;52:73.

49. Kaufman B: The turcica—A manifestation of the intrasellar subarachnoid space. Endocrinology 1968;90:931.

50. Jenkins JS, Gilbert J, Ang V: Hypothalamic-pituitary function in patients with craniopharyngiomas. J Clin Endocrinol Metab 1976;43:394.

51. Krauss CM, Turksoy NR, Atkins L, et al: Familial premature ovarian failure due to an interstitial deletion of the long arm of the X chromosome. N Eng J Med 1987;317:125.

52. Alper MM, Garner PR: Premature ovarian failure: Its relationship to autoimmune disease. Obstet Gynecol 1985;66:27.

53. Kaufman F, Kogut MD, Donnell GN, et al: Ovarian failure in galactosaemia. Lancet 1979;ii:737.

54. Barbieri RL, Smith S, Ryan KJ: The role of hyperinsulinemia in the pathogenesis of ovarian hyperandrogenism. Fertil Steril 1988;50:197.

55. Lobo RA, Kletzky OA, Campeau JD: Elevated bioactive luteinizing hormone in women with polycystic ovary syndrome. Fertil Steril 1983;39:674.

56. Yen SSC: The polycystic ovary syndrome. Clin Endocrinol 1980;12:177.

57. Lobo RA, Granger LR, Paul WL, et al: Psychological stress and increases in urinary norepinephrine metabolites, platelet sertotonin and adrenal androgens in women with polycystic ovary syndrome. Am J Obstet Gynecol 1983;145:495.

58. Yen SCC, Jaffe RB, eds. Reproductive endocrinology. Philadelphia: WB Saunders, 1986:456.

59. Tanabe K, Gagliano P, Channing CP, et al: Levels of inhibin-activity and steroids in human follicular fluid from normal women and women with polycystic ovarian disease. J Clin Endocrinol Metab 1983;57:24.

60. Barbieri RL, Ryan KJ: Hyperandrogenism, insulin resistence and acanthosis nigricans syndrome. A common endocrinopathy with distinct pathophysiological features. Am J Obstet Gynecol 1983;147:90.

61. Smith S, Ravnikar VA, Barbieri RL: Androgen and insulin response to an oral glucose challenge in hyperandrogenic women. Fertil Steril 1987;40:237.

62. Barbieri RL, Makris A, Ryan KJ: Effects of insulin on steroidogenesis in cultured porcine ovarian theca. Fertil Steril 1983;40:237.

63. Barbieri RL, Makris A. Randall RW, et al: Insulin stimulates androgen accumulation in incubations of ovarian stroma obtained from women with hyperandrogenism. J Clin Endocrinol Metab 1986;62:904.

64. Flier JS, Eastman RC, Minaker KL, et al: Acanthosis nigricans in obese women with hyperandrogenism. Diabetes 1985;34:101.

65. March CM, Israel R: Intrauterine adhesions secondary to elective abortion. Hysteroscopic diagnosis and management. Obstet Gynecol 1976;48:422.

CHAPTER 10

Abnormal Bleeding in the Adolescent Patient

Ann Jeanette Davis, MD

Appropriate central nervous system maturation at puberty culminates in normal menstrual function. Negative feedback between estrogen and follicle-stimulating hormone (FSH) and positive feedback between estrogen and luteinizing hormone (LH) results in a cyclic dynamic predictable pattern.

The proliferative phase of the menstrual cycle is associated with FSH stimulation of follicular growth and estradiol secretion. Estradiol stimulates an orderly growth and regeneration of endometrial tissue. At estradiol levels of 200 pg per milliliter sustained over 52 hours, the LH surge and ovulation occur (positive feedback).[2] Progesterone dominates the hormonal milieu in the second half of the menstrual cycle, known as the secretory phase. The endometrial tissue is stabilized by the antimitotic progesterone influence and readies itself for menstrual shedding. Declining levels of estrogen cause FSH to rise, leading to new follicular development and ongoing menstrual cycling (negative feedback). Normative data reveals ovulatory menstrual cycles may range between 21–40 days with 40–100 cc of flow.[3] Despite the 55–82% incidence of anovulatory cycles in the first menarcheal year,[4] most adolescents do not present with abnormal bleeding, as their flow patterns still fall within these acceptable normatives.

ABNORMAL MENSTRUAL FLOW

Abnormal menstrual bleeding may be divided into cyclic shedding with superimposed abnormal flow versus noncyclic anovulatory shedding, ie, recycling failure (see Table 10-1). The menstrual history, which is often

ISSN 1043-3198/89/$3.50

Clinical Practice of Gynecology: **3,** 120–130, 1989

Table 10-1. Abnormal Gynecologic Bleeding in Adolescent Patients

Differential Diagnoses	
Cyclic shedding with superimposed abnormal bleeding (Generally ovulatory)	Noncyclic shedding (recycling failure) (Anovulatory)

Pregnancy	

Blood dyscrasia	Endocrine
	  thyroid
	  Cushings
	  congenital adrenal hyperplasia
	  ovarian failure

Adeno-carcinoma vagina	

Anatomic
  trauma (foreign object, tampon)
  polyps
  myoma
  congenital malformation
  cervical hemangiomas
	Tumors
	  ovarian
	    Sertoli-Leydig granulosa
	    theca
	  prolactinoma

Infectious
  cervicitis
  PID (endometritis)
	Other
	  psychogenic/stress
	  exercise related
	  eating disorders
	  systemic disease

Other
  endometriosis
  midcycle ovulatory spotting	

Abnormal ovulatory cycles
  "nonclassical DUB"
  possible corpus luteum deficiency
  possible occult endometritis
	Chronic anovulation
	  "classical DUB"

difficult to obtain, is critical to help make this differentiation. The young woman who states she is having three periods a month may actually have 4 days of moderate flow associated with two other episodes of irregular spotting. A menstrual calendar with careful attention to the type of bleeding (quantity, coloration, duration) can prove to be an invaluable aid. However, perception of heavy blood loss is notoriously poor, especially among adolescent patients. Fraser[5] reports no correlation between the number of pads or tampons and measured blood loss. Forty-five percent of patients complaining of heavy menstrual flow actually had light-to-moderate loss. Conversely, perception of light blood loss tends to be very accurate.

Dysfunctional uterine bleeding (DUB) is traditionally defined as abnormal menstrual bleeding without any local or systemic cause. This term is widely used, misunderstood, and abused. Recycling failure, a more descriptive term, refers to interruption of the cycling mechanism, which is characteristic of the anovulatory cycle. The rare ovulatory DUB patient ("nonclassical DUB") may represent occult endometritis, corpus luteum deficiency, or other undefined etiologies. Only 10% of DUB patients are ovulatory.[6]

Division of irregular bleeding into noncyclic (anovulatory) bleeding versus cyclic shedding with superimposed abnormal bleeding directs the clinician toward proper treatment (see Table 10-1). For example, a patient with postcoital bleeding caused by cervicitis would present with regular menstrual flow and superimposed abnormal bleeding. If this patient were assumed to have noncyclic shedding (anovulation), she might be improperly treated with hormonal manipulation.

Anovulation leads to excessive bleeding because of interruption of the normal dynamic hormonal milieu. Absence of progesterone production from the corpus luteum prevents well-developed endometrial structural rigidity and development of the proper endometrial cleavage plane.[7] Vascular changes in chronic proliferative endometrium are not orderly, and breakdown may occur from the fluctuating estrogenic support. Unopposed estrogens result in large quantities of growth that must be desquamated. Bleeding is not a universal event, and a fragmentary endometrial shedding occurs.

DIFFERENTIAL DIAGNOSIS OF ABNORMAL BLEEDING IN THE ADOLESCENT

Pregnancy

Pregnancy must certainly be excluded in every adolescent presenting with abnormal bleeding. Seventy percent of adolescents have had intercourse prior to age 19, and only half of these use protection at the time of their first coitus.[8] Enzyme-linked immunoassays of urinary human chorionic gonadotrophin (hCG) are sensitive to approximately 50 mU/mL, signaling very early gestations.[9] These tests can be performed quickly using the patient's urine.

CYCLIC SHEDDING/OVULATORY

Blood Dyscrasias

Blood dyscrasias can often present with heavy menstrual flow. Claessens, in a study of 59 adolescents with menorrhagia, found a 20% incidence of blood dyscrasias.[10] Patients displaying severe menorrhagia at menarche had a 50% incidence of bleeding disorders (see Figures 10-1 and 10-2). A bleeding time is often overlooked but critical, as patients with von Willebrand's disease can present with normal coagulation studies. History of epistaxis, bleeding with tooth loss, and familial bleeding problems, or physical findings, including petechiae and excessive bruisability, may lead the physician to suspect strongly a blood dyscrasia. Patients with blood dys-

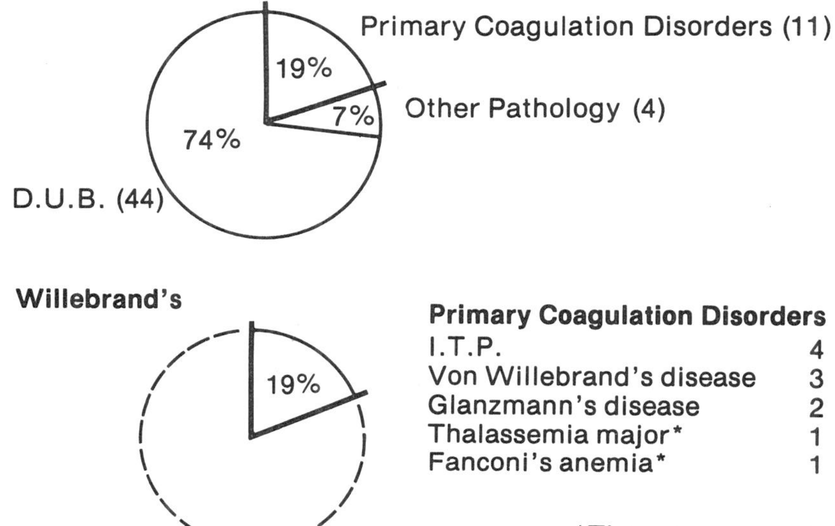

FIGURES 10-1, 10-2 Etiology of acute adolescent menorrhagia in 59 cases. From Claessens and Cowell: Acute adolescent menorrhagia. Am J Obstet Gynecol 1981; 139:278, with permission.

crasias tend to bleed regularly but with prolonged and heavy menstrual flows.

Adenocarcinoma of the Vagina

Abnormal bleeding may be a presenting symptom of adenocarcinoma of the vagina, a rare but aggressive cancer, which is found in .14–1.4/1000 diethylstilbestrol (DES)-exposed progeny.[11] Of the reported cases of adenocarcinoma, 25% do not have a history of maternal DES exposure.[3] Findings may include microscopic-to-large vaginal tumors that are polypoid, flat, or ulcerative in character.

Anatomic

Intermenstrual spotting and bleeding may signal the presence of cervical or endometrial polyps. Submucous myomas can also be seen in this age group, although they are rare. Myomas may present with increasing menstrual flow after the initial normal menstrual flow has slowed. Rarely, bleeding cervical hemangiomas may be the source of heavy vaginal bleeding.

Foul-smelling vaginal bleeding is often seen in the presence of a foreign object. Chronic bleeding vaginal ulcers resulting from daily tampon insertion have also caused abnormal menstrual patterns.

Congenital malformations, especially those with partial obstruction, can be easily misdiagnosed as dysfunctional uterine bleeding. These may present with vaginal or pelvic masses and prune colored bleeding following a normal menstrual flow.

Infectious/Other Causes

Endometriosis may present with dark-colored premenstrual spotting. Pelvic inflammatory disease can cause irregular spotting due to endometritis. Cervicitis and cervical polyps may result in irregular bleeding, which is often post-coital in character.

ANOVULATORY/NONCYCLIC SHEDDING

Endocrine

Recycling failure can be caused by endocrine disorders. Hypothyroidism may present with heavy prolonged menstrual bleeds, and hyperthyroidism may cause a wide spectrum of menstrual irregularities. Cushing's syndrome should be suspected in patients presenting with stria, hypertension, truncal obesity, and menstrual irregularity. Evidence of excessive androgenization, such as acne, clitoromegaly, hirsutism, and an abnormal menstrual pattern, may be evidence of congenital adrenal hyperplasia.

Ovarian failure can also first present with abnormal menstrual cycling. Five percent of Turner's patients presenting with delayed puberty have some menstrual shedding, and as many as 46% of chromosomally competent ovarian failures (46XX) patients have menstrual flow.[12]

Tumors

Prolactinomas prevent regular menstrual cycling via interruption of the pulsatile release of gonadotrophin-releasing hormone (GNRH) and inhibition of ovarian steroidogenesis. Galactorrhea is only displayed in one-third of patients with elevated prolactins.[2] A history of establishment of normal menstrual cycling followed by irregular cycling always makes a prolactinoma suspect. Prolactinomas have not been reported prior to puberty, as estrogen is apparently at least necessary for initial development of this tumor.

Menstrual irregularity may be the presenting complaint of patients with

Sertoli–Leydig or granulosa-theca cell tumors of the ovary secondary to tumor cell steroid production. These additional steroids interrupt normal menstrual cycling, creating anovulatory cycles. The majority of these patients have palpable masses on pelvic exam.[13]

Other Causes of Anovulatory Bleeding

Stress, resulting in anovulation, is a common cause of menstrual irregularity. Twenty-one percent of coeds entering Edinburgh University showed abnormal menstrual cycling in Sheldrake's study.[14] A similar percentage of women entering convents also display recycling failure prior to weight or activity changes.[15]

Strenuous athletic participation may be the cause of anovulation and irregular uterine bleeding. Fritch theorizes that a 20% ratio of body fat to body mass is critical for continued normal menstrual cycling.[16] In her study of 89 ballerinas, 12% had delayed menarche, 14% had amenorrhea, and 30% had irregular cycling.[17]

Body fat, however, does not appear to be the only critical factor, as swimmers involved in strenuous workouts with normal body fat also display menstrual irregularities.[18] This is probably secondary to stress causing hypothalamic depression of normal GNRH release.

Irregular menstrual cycling may be found during the evaluation and resolution of eating disorders. Severe eating disorder patients will progress to an amenorrheic state. Anorexics and bulemics may have loss of body fat or stress-associated hypothalamic suppression causing inappropriate GNRH release. Ten percent of anorexics who reattain normal body fat do not cycle normally, apparently secondary to hypothalamic suppression unrelated to body fat percentage.[19]

Systemic disease such as enteritis can also cause irregular cycling either due to less of body fat or stress.

Chronic Anovulation/"Classical DUB"

Although all the previously listed diagnostic possibilities must be considered, the major cause of abnormal uterine bleeding in adolescents is chronic anovulation from inappropriate maturation of the hypothalamic–ovarian axis. The normal dynamic hormonal milieu is absent, and only estrogenic support of the endometrium occurs.

EVALUATION AND TREATMENT OF IRREGULAR BLEEDING

Although the differential diagnosis of irregular bleeding is extensive, a history, physical, and limited lab work can usually exclude local or systemic

Table 10-2. Laboratory Studies to Exclude Local or Systemic Disease

Patient	Tests
All patients	Urine hCG CBC with platelets
Documented drop in HGB or HGB <10	Coagulation studies (PT/PTT) Bleeding time
As indicated	Thyroid function test, prolactin, ACTH stimulation test, overnight cortisol suppression, glucose, FSH/LH, progesterone, basal body temperature chart, Pap smear

Abbreviation: HGB, Hemoglobin.

disease (see Table 10-2). A complete blood count with platelets and a pregnancy test are standard routine laboratory studies. History and physical exam may indicate other appropriate evaluations. If local or systemic causes are identified, treatment to correct these is naturally indicated. Hormonal manipulation to effect hemostasis and prevent reoccurrences may be required in: 1) recycling failure and 2) blood dyscrasias. The degree of hemorrhage can be assessed from the physical exam and the patient's blood count.

Patients with hemoglobins less than 10 g/dL should be hospitalized (see Figure 10-3). In those with hemoglobins less than 10 g/dL and acute bleeding, hospitalization should be considered. In severe cases, 25–40 mg Premarin intravenously every 4 hours for a total of three to six dosages will control bleeding in over 70% of patients.[20] Intravenous Premarin has been found to be effective in treating bleeding secondary to a wide variety of biopsy-proven pathology, including secretory, proliferative, menstrual, and polypoid endometrium as well as endometritis.[20] A high progestational oral preparation must be given concurrently with the intravenous Premarin (such as Ovral or Norlutate). Appropriate dosages of these agents would be one, four times a day for 4 days; one, three times a day for 3 days; and one, twice a day for 2 weeks (see Figure 10-3). A schematic representation of this hormonal hemostasis can be found in Figure 10-4.

Studies indicate that progestational agents are more effective when combined with small dosages of estrogen.[3] Despite use of an antiemetic, some patients cannot tolerate oral estrogens. Oral progestational agents are appropriate in this group. However, in the patient with prolonged bleeding, or the patient postdilation and curettage, progesterones alone will often not be therapeutic. These patients have essentially no endometrium left for the progestin to stabilize.

Adolescents with hemoglobins less than 10 g/dL, especially those

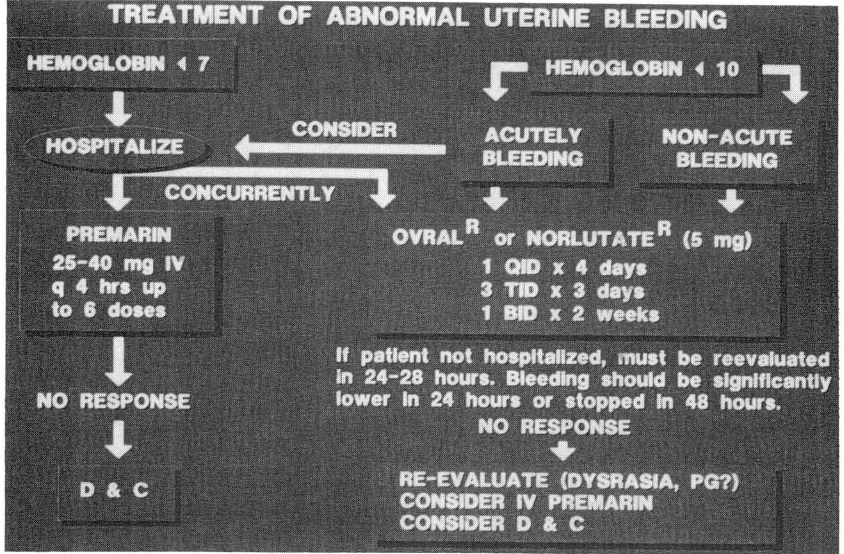

FIGURE 10-3 Treatment of abnormal uterine bleeding in the adolescent patient.

treated as an outpatient, require follow-up in 24–48 hours. Failure of the hormonal regimen should cause the clinician to reevaluate and make sure that a blood dyscrasia or pregnancy was not overlooked. Rarely, a dilation and curettage must be done to control adolescent bleeding.

Patients presenting with hemoglobins greater than 10 g/dL can generally be treated on an outpatient basis. In acute bleeds, the same Ovral or Norlutate regimen may be employed. Patients without a significant hemoglobin decrease can be managed by Ovral, one tablet four times a day for 5 days followed by a withdrawal bleed.[3] Teenagers may be discouraged by this regimen, as a relatively heavy withdrawal bleed will occur. However, this regimen is easy for the adolescent to remember and gains her confidence that the clinician does have something to stop her bleeding.

Adolescents treated for irregular bleeding should be cycled for at least 3 months. If after 3 months, contraception is not required, the patient can be given a trial off hormones to determine if cycling will recur. If cycling does not occur, the patient should be artificially cycled. Appropriate medications to induce this withdrawal include 10 mg Provera for 12 days each month or use of oral contraceptives.

Patients with mild menstrual irregularities can often be given reassurance, a menstrual calendar, and followed carefully. Early menarche results in quicker establishment of ovulatory cycles and earlier establishment of regular cycling. The interval of time from menarche until 50% of cycles are ovulatory is 1, 3, and 4.5 years when menarche is

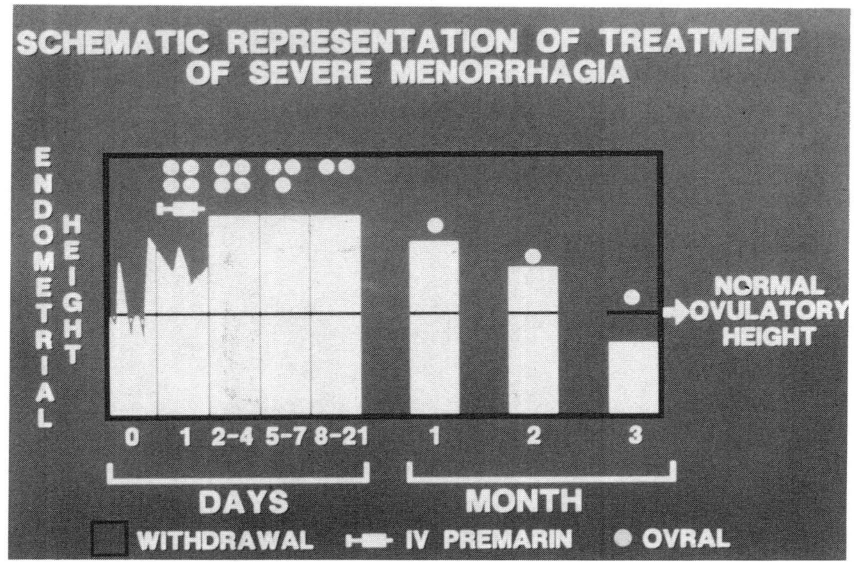

FIGURE 10-4 Schematic treatment of severe recycling failure in the adolescent patient. Adapted from Claessens and Cowell: Acute adolescent menorrhagia. Am J Obstet Gynecol 1981; 139:278.

less than 12 years, 12–12.9 years, and 13 or more years, respectively.[21] If adolescents do not establish regular cycling within a reasonable variation from the above normatives, hormonal therapy should be considered. Adolescents may use mild menstrual abnormalities as their ticket to the gynecologist's office in hopes of obtaining contraception. This possibility should always be explored.

Iron therapy should be initiated to raise blood counts if appropriate. Acute bleeders receiving high-dose estrogens may not tolerate iron therapy initially secondary to gastric distress from both iron and estrogens. Antiprostaglandins appear to decrease menstrual flow and are also appropriate in some cases.

CONCLUSION

The assumption that all cases of adolescent menstrual irregularity are "classical DUB" can cause clinicians to overlook local and systemic pathology. Both the ovulatory and anovulatory bleeder may have an identifiable etiology of their problem. Adolescents presenting with abnormal gynecologic bleeding deserve a thoughtful evaluation. Abnormal bleeding can be divided into cyclic shedding with superimposed abnormal bleeding (generally ovulatory) and noncyclic shedding or recycling failure (anovulatory) (see Table 10-1). Recycling failure may be due to systemic causes or "classical DUB."

The long-term prognosis of adolescents presenting with anovulatory bleeding is discouraging. Southam and Richart[22] reported continued bleeding problems in 50% of women 4 years after their initial presentation. Noncycling women are at high risk for serious gynecologic morbidity, including infertility and endometrial cancer. Emphasis should be placed on careful long-term surveillance with the use of progestational agents to prevent serious endometrial pathology in these noncycling women.

REFERENCES

1. Kuvin SF: Near-fatal menarche. Clin Pediatr 1964;3:177.
2. Speroff L, Glass RH, Kase NG: Clinical gynecologic endocrinology and infertility. Baltimore: Williams and Wilkins, 1983:225–243.
3. Altchek A: Dysfunctional uterine bleeding in adolescence. Clin Obstet Gynecol 1977;20:633.
4. Gantt PA, McDonough PG: Dysfunctional bleeding in adolescents. In Barwin BN and Belisle S, eds. Adolescent gynecology and sexuality. New York: Masson Publishing USA Inc, 1982:59–78.
5. Fraser IS: A preliminary study of factors influencing perception of menstrual blood loss volume. Am J Obstet Gynecol 1984;149:788.
6. Jones GS: Endocrine problems of the adolescent. Md Med J 1967;16:45.
7. Stricker RC: Dysfunctional uterine bleeding: Diagnosis and treatment. Postgrad Med J 1979;66:135.
8. Alan Guttmacher Institute: Teenage pregnancy: The problem that hasn't gone away. New York: AGI, 1981.
9. Emancipator K, Cadoff EM, Burke MD: Analytical versus clinical sensitivity and specificity in pregnancy testing. Am J Obstet Gynecol 1988;158:613.
10. Claessens E, Cowell C: Dysfunctional uterine bleeding in the adolescent. Pediatr Clin North Am 1981;28:369.
11. Herbst AL: Clear cell adenocarcinoma and current status of DES-exposed females. Cancer 1981;48:484.
12. Reindollar RH, Byrd JR, McDonough PG: Delayed sexual development: A study of 252 patients. Am J Obstet Gynecol 1981;14:371.
13. Huffman JW, Dewhurst CJ, Capraro VJ: The gynecology of childhood and adolescence. Philadelphia: WB Saunders, 1981:297–307.
14. Sheldrake P, Cormach M: Variation in menstrual cycle symptoms reporting. J Pschosom Res 1976;20:169.
15. Drew FL, Stifel EN: Secondary amenorrhea among young women entering religious life. Obstet Gynecol 1968;32:47.
16. Frisch RE, McArthur JW: Menstrual cycles: Fatness as a determinant of minimum weight for height for their maintenance or onset. Science 1974;185:949.
17. Frisch RE, Wyshaht D, Vincent C: Delayed menarche and amenorrhea in ballet dancers. N Engl J Med 1980;303:17.
18. Frisch RE, Johnson TS, Marion BJ, et al: Secondary amenorrhea in athletes. Lancet 1978;ii:1145.
19. Hsu L, Cripst AH, Harding B: Outcome of anorexia nervosa. Lancet 1979;i:61–65.

20. DeVore GR, Owens O, Kase N: Use of intraveneous premarin in the treatment of dysfunctional uterine bleeding—a double blind randomized control study. Obstet Gynecol 1982;59:285.
21. Apter D, Vihko R: Early menarche, a risk factor for breast cancer, indicates early onset of ovulatory cycles. J Clin Endocrinol Metab 1983;57:82.
22. Southam A, Richart R: The prognosis for adolescents with menstrual abnormalities. Am J Obstet Gynecol 1966;94:637.

CHAPTER 11

Management of Breast Masses in Adolescent Females

Donald Peter Goldstein, MD, and
Odette Pinsonneault, MD

Breast masses occur infrequently in adolescent females and often pose a problem in management. Virtually all breast masses are either benign tumors or physiologic swellings that regress spontaneously. Although malignancy is rare, patients and parents are concerned about any breast abnormalities and the cosmetic aspects of breast surgery. These issues must be taken into consideration when one is confronted with this problem.

This chapter summarizes the experiences with adolescent female breast masses accumulated over a period of 11 years by the Division of Gynecology at The Children's Hospital. Based on this data, a clinical approach to the problem, surgical indications, and some technical considerations are suggested.

MATERIALS AND METHODS

Between January 1972 and December 1983, 86 female adolescents were operated upon for persistent or enlarging breast masses. Patients who presented with a breast mass were examined by a staff gynecologist. Puncture aspiration was performed on all cystic masses. When fluid was obtained, no surgery was performed. Mammograms were not obtained. Surgery was recommended when the mass was firm, not decompressable, persistent, or enlarging. Operations were carried out on an ambulatory or inpatient basis depending on the medical status of the patient. All pathology specimens were reviewed by the Department of Pathology, The Children's Hospital.

Clinical Practice of Gynecology: **3,** 131–136, 1989
© 1989 Elsevier Science Publishing Co., Inc.
655 Avenue of the Americas, New York, NY 10010

131

ISSN 1043-3198/89/$3.50

Table 11-1. Summary of 102 Breast Procedures in 86 Adolescent Females

	N	(%)
Type of surgery		
Excisional biopsy	99	(91)
Incision and drainage	1	(1)
Incision and drainage and excisional biopsy	1	(1)
Needle aspiration	1	(1)
Repeated procedures	16	(16)
Two procedures: 13 (15% of patients)		
Four procedures: 1 (1% of patients)		
Site of lesion		
Unilateral	91	(89)
Bilateral	11	(11)
Hospital status		
Ambulatory	97	(95)
Inpatient	5	(5)
Type of anesthesia		
General	74	(73)
Local	28	(27)
Type of incision		
Circumareolar	52	(51)
Curvilinear	30	(29)
Unspecified	20	(20)

RESULTS

A total of 102 surgical procedures were performed in 86 patients, who ranged in age from 8 to 19 years (mean: 16.3 years). Table 11–1 summarizes the details of these procedures. In the majority of the patients, surgery consisted of excisional biopsy. Fourteen patients underwent repeat procedures for recurrence. Bilateral lesions were present in 11% of patients. Only five procedures were done on an inpatient basis—two because of an intercurrent medical condition, two because of the size of the mass, and one because of associated inflammatory signs. General anesthesia was used in approximately three-quarters of the patients. The lesion was excised through a circumareolar incision in 51% of cases. During the last year of the study, this type of incision was utilized in 70% of the procedures. There were no operative complications.

The pathologic diagnosis of 100 biopsy specimens are listed in Table 11–2. The two patients who underwent incision and drainage and needle aspiration respectively are excluded because no pathologic specimen was obtained. No malignant disease was encountered. Fibroadenoma was the predominant pathologic finding (83%).

Table 11-2.

	N (pct)
Fibroadenoma	
Adult	58
Juvenile	19
Giant	2
Cellular	2
Papillary	1
Fibroadenoma with mixed stroma	1
Total	83 (83)
Fibrocystic mastopathy	
Fibrocystic disease	5
Simple cyst	2
Stromal sclerosis	1
Total	8 (8)
Other	
Chronic mastitis	2
Epidermal inclusion cyst	1
Adenomatous hyperplasia	1
Intraductal hyperplasia with focal secretion	1
Capillary hemangioma	1
Fat necrosis	1
Normal fat and breast tissue	1
Total	9 (9)

DISCUSSION

The results of this study confirm the previously reported high incidence of fibroadenomas and the rarity of malignancy associated with breast masses in adolescent females.[1] Although they are extremely rare, malignant tumors do occur in adolescents. Farrow and Ashikari[2] reported one case of primary breast carcinoma among 237 patients aged 10–20 years, for an incidence of 0.4%. Haagensen[3] reported that 0.02% of breast carcinomas were found in women younger than 25 years of age. In the study by Norris and Taylor[4] of 5,000 cases of breast cancer, 23 patients (0.46%) were under 25 years of age while one (0.02%) was under 20. Mammography has not proven to be of great value in this age group and is rarely indicated.

All physicians dealing with adolescent females should be familiar with the physiology of breast development. Very often, a premenarchal patient is seen because of the presence of a unilateral or bilateral tender subareolar mass. In these circumstances, the normally developing breast bud should be recognized. It is a firm, button-shaped structure approximately 1 cm in diameter. Excision or biopsy will lead to dramatic and inexcusable iatrogenic amastia or breast deformity.

In general, pathologic masses are eccentric in location. Fibroadenomas

Table 11-3. Surgical Indications in Adolescent Breast Masses

1. Persistent breast mass
2. Rapidly growing mass
3. Presence of abnormal cells on cyst aspirate
4. Recurrence of cystic mass after aspiration
5. Nipple discharge
6. Patient's anxiety

are characterized by the presence of an asymptomatic, firm, rubbery, mobile mass sometimes irregular in shape that may vary in size from a few millimeters to many centimeters and may be multiple and bilateral. In fibrocystic disease, cysts tend to be tender and to vary in size and location with menstrual cycles. These patients should be placed on a caffeine-free diet. Brooks and colleagues[5] demonstrated an 88% improvement in symptoms, a 91% reduction in palpable nodularities, and an 85% improvement in graphic thermal patterns after 6 months of caffeine restriction in patients with fibrocystic breast disease. A cystic mass should be aspirated using a 23-g needle. This procedure is usually well tolerated by adolescents and does not necessitate anesthesia. Very often, the cyst collapses following this procedure and does not recur. All fluid obtained should be sent for cytologic examination, and the patient should be observed carefully in order to diagnose any recurrence.

It is certainly advisable to observe a breast mass in an adolescent for three to six menstrual cycles. This allows some masses to regress spontaneously and avoids unnecessary procedures. Furnival and colleagues[6] demonstrated the accuracy of clinical diagnosis in 70 women aged 17–25 years presenting with breast symptoms. By the application of a conservative approach, fewer than half of their patients with palpable mass on initial examination eventually needed biopsy because of persistence.

Indications for surgical excision are summarized in Table 11–3. All persistent or rapidly growing masses should be excised, since it is the only accurate means of obtaining a definite diagnosis. Furthermore, even though benignity is almost certain, the presence of a persistent mass is a tremendous source of anxiety for the patient, which in itself represents a sufficient surgical indication in this age group. The presence of nipple discharge is also an indication for surgery because of its possible association with an intraductal papilloma, cystosarcoma phylloides, or other malignant lesions.

When one is proceeding with surgery, consideration should be given to the cosmetic results. In the recent years, we have tried to excise as many masses as possible through circumareolar incisions that result in almost invisible scars. It is generally accepted that one-half of the areolar circumference can be incised without compromising the blood supply. Even when located quite far from the areola, it is usually possible to reach the mass by raising an areolar flap and dissecting under the skin. The utilization of the electrocautery for dissection and meticulous hemostasis reduces the risk of postoperative hematomas. A small penrose drain may be utilized when necessary. In our experience, fibroadenomas as large as 10 × 10 cm can be excised through this type of incision without complications. When the circumareolar route is judged unacceptable because of the size or location of the mass, efforts should be made to respect the natural skin folds and avoid radial incisions. The defect created in the deep breast tissue should be carefully closed in order to avoid postoperative deformity. For skin closure, a fine subcuticular suture gives good results. However, because the curvature of the circumareolar incision makes perfect approximation of the skin difficult, we feel that the utilization of interrupted 4-0 nylon sutures that are removed on the third or fourth postoperative day gives the best cosmetic results.

It is to be remembered that fibroadenomas frequently prove to be either lobulated or larger than they appear at the time of preoperative palpation. Therefore, careful palpation of the surrounding breast tissue should be carried out after excision to ensure that lobules of the lesion are not left behind.

The vast majority of breast procedures in adolescents can be carried out on an ambulatory basis, which is certainly less emotionally disturbing and expensive for the patient. The choice of anesthesia depends on the individual adolescent's ability to cooperate and on the extent of the dissection that will be required. In young patients where the anesthetic risk is usually very low, it seems preferable to proceed under general anesthesia through a circumareolar incision than to sacrifice the cosmetic result by using a more direct peripheral incision under local anesthesia.

Although the pathologic diagnosis of an adolescent breast mass does not usually create any therapeutic controversy, the surgeon should be careful in interpreting a pathologic report mentioning *c. phylloides.* As mentioned by Oberman,[7] this term suggesting the presence of a malignant tumor is, in fact, utilized to describe a wide variety of benign and malignant lesions ranging from cellular juvenile fibroadenoma to fibrosarcoma. Therefore, this pathologic diagnosis should always prompt a pathology consultation in order to avoid over- or underinterpretation.

Finally, an article on breast masses would not be complete without a few words about self-examination. Hein and colleagues[8] reported that of 95 teenagers admitted for a breast mass, 77 (81%) had been self-detected. Although in this study it was not known whether the patients had been previously instructed in breast self-examination, this certainly proves that adolescents are concerned with their own health and that teaching them breast self-examination is worth the effort.

REFERENCES

1. Goldstein DP, Miller V: Breast masses in adolescent females. Clin Pediatr 1982;21:17.
2. Farrow JH, Ashikari H: Breast lesions in young girls. Surg Clin North Am 1969;49:261.
3. Haagensen CD: Diseases of the breast. Philadelphia: WB Saunders, 1974.
4. Norris HJ, Taylor HB: Carcinoma of the breast in women less than thirty years old. Cancer 1970;26:953.
5. Brooks PG, Gait S, Heldfond AJ, Margolin ML, Allen AS: Measuring the effect of caffeine restriction on fibrocystic breast disease. J Reprod Med 1981;26:279.
6. Furnival CM, Irwin JRM, Gray GM: Breast disease in young women: When is biopsy indicated? Med J Aust 1983;2:167.
7. Oberman HA: Breast lesions in the adolescent female. Pathol Annu 1979;14:175.
8. Hein K, Dell R, Cohen M: Self-detection of a breast mass in adolescent females. J Adolesc Health Care 1982;3:15.

CHAPTER 12

Pelvic Pain in the Pediatric and Adolescent Patient

Donald Peter Goldstein, MD, and
Odette Pinsonneault, MD

Acute and chronic pelvic pain accounts for a substantial number of office and emergency ward consultations for the gynecologists who deal with the adolescent age group. The reasons are twofold: First, there is a tendency to attribute all pain "below the umbilicus" in peri- and postmenarchal females to a gynecologic etiology; second, most physicians are reluctant to perform a pelvic examination in the young patient.

The differential diagnosis of pelvic pain, in fact, includes a wide variety of gynecologic, nongynecologic and functional or psychosomatic causes. The purpose of this chapter is to suggest an efficient approach to this common and challenging problem.

ACUTE PELVIC PAIN

Acute pelvic pain necessitates aggressive management because of the intensity of symptoms and the possibility that a potentially life-threatening condition may exist.

Differential Diagnosis

The differential of acute pelvic pain in adolescents is summarized in Table 12-1. The gynecologic causes can be divided into three categories: infection, rupture, and torsion. In general, symptoms associated with infection usually develop progressively over a few days. In cases of rupture or torsion, pain occurs suddenly, and the patient can most often tell precisely at what time symptoms began. Nongynecologic etiologies involve mainly the digestive or the urinary tract.

Clinical Practice of Gynecology: **3**, 137–145, 1989
© 1989 Elsevier Science Publishing Co., Inc.
655 Avenue of the Americas, New York, NY 10010

ISSN 1043-3198/89/$3.50

Table 12-1. Differential Diagnosis of Acute Pelvic Pain in Adolescent Females

Gynecologic causes
  Infection
    Pelvic inflammatory disease
  Rupture
    Follicular cyst
    Corpus luteum cyst
    Endometrioma
    Tumor
  Torsion
    Ovarian cyst
    Tube
    Hydatid of Morgagni

Nongynecologic causes
  Gastrointestinal
    Appendicitis
    Mechel diverticulitis
    Gastroenteritis
    Mesenteric adenitis
    Intestinal obstruction
  Urinary
    Cystitis
    Pyelonephritis
    Calculi

History and Physical Examination

The history should define, as exactly as possible, the sequence of events, the pain location and its radiation, and associated gastrointestinal, urinary tract, and systemic symptoms. A careful menstrual, contraceptive, and sexual history is also mandatory.

A complete physical examination should, of course, be performed. Special attention is paid to the abdomen to localize the pain, define the presence of, and identify peritoneal signs and evidence of bowel obstruction. A pelvic exam must be performed on every patient in order to determine the uterine size, shape and symmetry, the presence of adnexal or cervical tenderness, and to identify adnexal masses or thickening.

Diagnostic Studies

The basic laboratory workup should include a complete blood count with differential, an erythrocyte sedimentation rate, a complete urinalysis, a urine culture, a pregnancy test, and a cervical culture for gonococcus and chlamydia.

The finding of a high white count and/or sedimentation rate suggests the presence of either an infectious or inflammatory process, or the presence of ischemia, usually secondary to adnexal torsion or bowel obstruction. Hemoglobin and hematocrit are usually poor indicators of bleeding, since in acute hemorrhage, hemodilution may not have occurred. Depending on the type of pregnancy test utilized, it should be remembered that a negative result does not always rule out early intrauterine or an ectopic pregnancy.

A pelvic ultrasound may be valuable to confirm the presence of a mass when the pelvic examination is not completely satisfactory, to identify the presence of free fluid in the cul-de-sac and to localize a suspected pregnancy.

Management

After these first steps have been taken, all patients fall into one of the following clinical categories:

1. There is a definite surgical emergency that necessitates immediate attention. In this situation, the suspected diagnosis is usually an acute hemoperitoneum, a ruptured tubo-ovarian abscess, an acute or ruptured appendicitis, or some other gastrointestinal surgical emergency.
2. The patient is suffering from a medical condition and adequate treatment is started (eg, urinary tract infection, gastroenteritis, pelvic inflammatory disease, etc).
3. The problem needs further investigation (eg, urinary calculi).
4. The condition remains undiagnosed and the question usually is "Does this patient have a pelvic inflammatory disease (PID), an ectopic pregnancy, appendicitis, or a ruptured or torsioned ovarian cyst?"

At this point, laparoscopy becomes an invaluable diagnostic tool. The potential risk of a surgical diagnostic procedure remains a concern for many physicians. In fact, a laparoscopy provides an immediate diagnosis that allows for appropriate medical or surgical treatment. It is also more cost-effective to perform an immediate laparoscopy than to subject the patient to a long period of inpatient observation, during which a surgical catastrophe, such as a ruptured appendicitis or ectopic pregnancy, remains a possibility. In cases of ruptured ovarian cysts or hemorrhagic corpus luteum, in which there is a no more active bleeding, it is possible to aspirate free blood and clots and ensure hemostasis by fulguration of bleeders. This technique may save the patient several days of agonizing pain and usually allows her to be discharged within 12 hours of the procedure.

In our judgment, the advantages of laparoscopy certainly outweigh the minimal surgical risk in these generally healthy teenagers, particularly where appendicitis is a real possibility.

Table 12-2 summarizes the principle laparoscopic diagnosis in 121

Table 12-2. Principal Laparoscopic Diagnoses in 121 Adolescent Females 11–17 Years Old with Acute Pelvic Pain*

	Patients	%
Ovarian cyst	47	39
Acute PID	21	17
Adnexal torsion	9	8
Endometriosis	6	5
Ectopic pregnancy	4	3
Appendicitis	13	11
No pathology	21	17

*The Children's Hospital, Boston; 1980–1986.
Abbreviation: PID, pelvic inflammatory disease.

patients ages 11–17 who presented at Boston Children's Hospital with acute abdominal pain between 1980 and 1986. In general, the most common cause of pain was due to some complication of an ovarian cyst. It is of interest that the causes of acute abdominal pain in the adolescent do not appear to be age related (Table 12-3).

CHRONIC PELVIC PAIN

Chronic pelvic pain (CPP) in adolescents is a frequent complaint and source of frustration for the patient, her parents, and her physician. It can be defined as 3 months or more of constant or intermittent, cyclic or acyclic pelvic pain, which has necessitated at least three separate visits to a physician without a definite diagnosis. Symptoms can be characterized by dull or severe pain, dysmenorrhea, dyspareunia, or vaginal pain. Very often these teenagers have been absent from school frequently, have seen a number of physicians, have undergone a number of radiologic examinations, and have tried a variety of analgesics without success. Many have already been referred for psychologic or psychiatric evaluation.

Guzenski[3] has drawn an excellent picture of the CPP patient with whom it is sometimes difficult to deal. After having been told, often more than once, that nothing is wrong with her, she may come to the physician with a considerable amount of anger, frustration, or desperation. Therefore, it is important to assure her that all efforts will be made to sort out her problem and that she will not be abandoned or her symptoms discussed as merely psychosomatic.

Differential Diagnosis

Table 12-4 summarizes the differential diagnosis of CPP in adolescent females. It includes many organ systems that can be responsible for pelvic

Table 12-3. Age Related Prevalence of Principal Laparoscopic Findings in 121 Adolescent Females 11–17 Years Old with Acute Pelvic Pain*

	Patients (%)		
	Age 11–13	Age 14–15	Age 16–17
Ovarian cyst	12 (50)	16 (35)	19 (37)
Acute PID	4 (17)	7 (16)	10 (19)
Adnexal torsion	0 (0)	7 (16)	2 (4)
Endometriosis	0 (0)	2 (4)	4 (7)
Ectopic pregnancy	0 (0)	3 (7)	1 (2)
Appendicitis	3 (13)	4 (9)	6 (12)
No pathology	5 (20)	6 (13)	10 (19)
Total	24 (20)	45 (37)	52 (43)

*The Children's Hospital, Boston: 1980–1986.
Abbreviation: PID, pelvic inflammatory disease.

symptoms either directly or by referred pain, as well as those of functional or psychogenic etiology.

An efficient approach to the problem depends on taking a thorough history and performing an adequate physical examination as well as with the judicious use of diagnostic studies.

History and Physical Examination

It is essential to review the complete history of the problem, including description, location and radiation of the pain, exacerbating and relieving factors, association with the menstrual cycle or with gastrointestinal, urinary, and musculoskeletal symptoms. The past medical and surgical history may also provide a clue. All prior diagnostic procedures and trials of treatment should be recorded, and, when possible, old medical records obtained. The familial and social history, as well as the association of the pain episodes with stressful events, should be detailed.

A complete physical examination should be performed, the abdomen being carefully palpated in search of any masses, tender areas, and organomegaly. Special care should be taken to differentiate deep pain from abdominal wall tenderness, especially in patients who have undergone prior surgeries where adhesions to the abdominal wall scar may be present. A skeletal assessment to identify any orthopedic abnormality that may be the cause of referred pelvic pain or associated with a congenital reproductive tract anomaly is also of great importance. A speculum examination should be performed to identify any vaginal or cervical anomaly and obtain cultures and cytology specimens. The bimanual recto–vaginal–abdominal palpation evaluates the pelvic structures and localizes tender areas. The posterior cul-de-sac should also be assessed for pain and nodularity.

Table 12-4. Differential Diagnosis of Chronic Pelvic Pain in Adolescent Females

Gynecologic causes
  Dysmenorrhea (primary, secondary)
  Mittelschmertz
  Endometriosis
  Chronic pelvic inflammatory disease
  Ovarian cyst
  Genital tract malformations
  Pelvic congestion
  Pelvic serositis

Gastrointestinal causes
  Constipation, bowel spasms
  Appendiceal fecaliths
  Bowel inflammatory diseases
  Dietary intolerance (lactose)

Urinary causes
  Urinary tract infection
  Hydranephrosis
  Urethral structure
  Urethral caruncle
  Urinary retention

Orthopedic causes
  Lordosis, kyphosis, scoliosis
  Herniation of intervertebral disk

Adhesions
  Postoperative
  Postpelvic infection

Psychogenic

Diagnostic Studies

The minimal laboratory workup in these patients consists of a complete blood count with differential and erythrocytic sedimentation rate, a urine analysis and culture, and cervical cultures for gonococcus and chlamydia. Other hematologic and biochemical studies are ordered, depending on clinical indications.

Pelvic ultrasonography may be useful to define a mass, provide information about a suspected genital tract malformation, and to screen patients in whom a satisfactory pelvic examination is impossible. Routine sonography in every patient is probably not advisable. In a study of 96 adolescents evaluated for CPP at The Cleveland Clinic, Gidwani[1] reported that of 15 patients in whom a pelvic mass was detected by ultrasound, only five were confirmed by laparoscopy.

No specific rules can be given regarding radiologic exams. It is certainly not advisable to submit all these teenagers to pelvic radiations without clinical indications. Gastrointestinal, urologic, and orthopedic studies should be ordered on the basis of the diagnostic impression after a thorough history and physical and laboratory workup are completed.

Laparoscopy

Laparoscopy is an invaluable tool to the diagnosis of CPP. It can diagnose or confirm the presence of organic disease that cannot be demonstrated by physical, radiologic, and sonographic examination. It allows the obtaining of appropriate biopsies and the performing of some primary therapy, such as fulguration of endometriosis, lysis of ahesions, and aspiration of ovarian cysts. Negative findings at laparoscopy may be equally valuable in reassuring the patient that no organic disease is present and help her accept the idea that she might have a functional problem that requires medical or emotional treatment.

Indications for laparoscopy in the evaluation of adolescents with CPP can be summarized as follows:

1. Dysmenorrhea unresponsive to the usual therapy with prostaglandin-inhibitors and/or ovulation suppression.
2. Confirmation or exclusion of clinically suspected endometriosis, chronic pelvic inflammatory disease, pelvic adhesions, appendiceal fecaliths, ovarian cyst and pelvic serositis.
3. Evaluation of undiagnosed pain after appropriate workup.

At Boston's Children's Hospital, our experience with laparoscopy in the diagnosis of CPP in adolescent females revealed that between July 1974 and December 1983, 282 patients ranging in age from 9 to 21 years underwent a diagnostic laparoscopy because of chronic pelvic symptoms.[2] Most of these adolescents had been referred to our gynecology service after a negative gastrointestinal and urinary tract workup or because of dysmenorrhea unresponsive to the usual therapy with prostaglandin inhibitors or oral contraceptives. Many of these patients had undergone psychiatric evaluation because of persistent and undiagnosed pain. Cases of chronic pelvic inflammatory disease were not included in the data because this condition is usually suspected on the basis of the past history and the finding of an elevated erythrocyte sedimentation rate. In these patients, a laparoscopy is usually performed to confirm the diagnosis and evaluate its severity rather than to establish the etiology of CPP.

All laparoscopies were performed under general endotracheal anesthesia, either on an inpatient or ambulatory basis. A uterine mobilizer was attached to the cervix to permit mobilization of the uterus. Approximately 2 L of carbon dioxide was utilized to create a pneumoperitoneum, and a 7-mm Wolf or Stortz laparoscope was introduced through an infraumbilical

Table 12-5. Postoperative Diagnosis in 282 Adolescent Females with Chronic Pelvic Pain*

	No. of Patients (%)
Endometriosis	126 (45)
Postoperative adhesions	37 (13)
Serositis	15 (5)
Ovarian cyst	14 (5)
Uterine malformation	15 (5)
Others†	4 (2)
No pathology	71 (25)

*The Children's Hospital, Boston: 1974–1983.
†Ileitis, infarcted hydatid of Morgagni, pelvic congestion.

incision. A second trocar site was established in the suprapubic area to allow the utilization of a probe or of a biopsy forceps.

Table 12-5 summarizes the postoperative diagnosis in these patients. Three-quarters of the patients were found to have intrapelvic pathology. Endometriosis was the most frequent finding, being diagnosed in 45% of cases. In most instances, the disease was mild to moderate, with implants located in the posterior cul-de-sac, on the ovaries, and on the lateral pelvic side walls. The next most common finding was postoperative adhesions, which was present in 13% of patients and were, for the most part, secondary to appendectomy or ovarian cystectomy.

One of the most puzzling laparoscopic findings was the presence of a pelvic serositis in 5% of the patients. This was characterized by hyperemia and granuloma-like lesions of the pelvic peritoneum and uterine serosa. Peritoneal biopsies revealed the presence of mesothelial hyperplasia with hemosiderin deposits. Peritoneal culture and cytology were normal. The significance of these changes remains unclear. It is the appearance of very early endometriosis, a reaction to repeated hemoperitoneum secondary to leaking corpus luteum or hemoperitoneum, a viral infection, or an incidental finding. These patients are very difficult to treat. Because of the small number of cases, no uniform therapy has emerged. Some patients respond to therapy with long-term prostaglandin inhibitors, others to ovulation suppression, and others to steroids. Long-term follow-up will hopefully better define this entity. A few patients with this finding have since developed endometriosis, confirmed at subsequent laparoscopy.

Other findings included ovarian cysts, uterine malformations of the obstructive type, cases of ileitis, infarcted hydatid of Morgagni, and pelvic congestion.

No organic disease was documented in 25% of the patients. In this group, pain was attributed to functional bowel disease or to psychogenic factors. Despite apparently normal bowel function, many teenagers with CPP improve when they are placed on a regimen of stool softeners and

Table 12-6. Age-related Incidence of Laparoscopic Findings in 129 Adolescent Females with Chronic Pelvic Pain*

	Number of Patients (%)				
	Age 11–13	Age 14–15	Age 16–17	Age 18–19	Age 20–21
Endometriosis	2 (12)	9 (28)	21 (40)	17 (45)	7 (54)
Postoperative adhesions	1 (6)	4 (13)	7 (13)	5 (13)	2 (15)
Serositis	5 (29)	4 (13)	0 (0)	2 (5)	0 (0)
Ovarian cyst	2 (12)	2 (6)	3 (5)	2 (5)	0 (8)
Uterine malformation	1 (6)	0 (0)	1 (2)	0 (0)	1 (0)
Others	0 (0)	1 (3)	2 (4)	1 (3)	0 (0)
No pathology	6 (35)	12 (37)	19 (36)	11 (29)	3 (23)

*The Children's Hospital, Boston: 1980–1983.

increased dietary fiber and fluid intake. The value of a negative laparoscopy should not be underestimated. In many instances, the assurance that their pelvic structures are normal is sufficient to improve the symptoms in these adolescents. Goldstein et al[2] reported that 74% of these patients were symptomatically improved after a negative laparoscopy. In a small number of these teenagers, adjunctive psychologic or behavioral modification therapy is necessary.

For the years 1980–1983, the results were broken down into age groups (Table 12-6). It is interesting to note that the incidence of endometriosis among adolescents complaining of CPP increases progressively with age, from 12% in the 11–13-year-old group to 54% in patients aged 20 and 21 years. Pelvic serositis, on the other hand, was encountered mostly in the 11–15-year-old group. Other findings remained fairly constant in all age groups.

SUMMARY

Acute and chronic pelvic pain in the adolescent patient needs to be taken seriously. In a vast majority of cases, an underlying cause can be identified. Under no circumstances should the label of psychogenic pain be offered on these teenagers without a prior negative laparoscopy. Adequate diagnosis and early therapy are essential in order to improve the quality of life and preserve the reproductive prognosis in these young patients.

REFERENCES

1. Gidwani GP: Laparoscopy for diagnosis of chronic pelvic pain. Transitions 1981:December.
2. Goldstein DP, DeCholnoky C, Emans SJ, et al: Laparoscopy in the diagnosis and management of pelvic pain in adolescents. J Reprod Med 1980;24:251.
3. Guzenski G: A new approach to chronic pelvic pain: The female patient. 1983;8:32/43.

CHAPTER 13

Congenital Anomalies in the Pediatric and Adolescent Female

Donald Peter Goldstein, MD, Odette Pinsonneault, MD, and Ann Jeanette Davis, MD

A large proportion of congenital abnormalities of the female genital tract remain undiscovered until adolescence. These are usually diagnosed when symptoms occur, especially menstrual disorders and coital difficulties, or simply because most patients undergo their first pelvic examination at this time. Those that are recognized in the infant and young child are external and usually noted either by a parent or the pediatrician.

Although some congenital malformations become obvious at first glance, the diagnosis of many of these defects requires a high index of suspicion. A thorough understanding of the nature of these anomalies is essential to gynecologists who deal with the teenage group. Early diagnosis, adequate treatment and appropriate psychologic support and counseling, assure the preservation of reproductive function when feasible and allows these adolescents to develop a serene attitude toward their sexuality.

CONGENITAL ANOMALIES IN PREPUBERTAL AGE GROUP

The most common abnormality seen in the neonate and young child is a cystic mass at the introitus. This is first observed in the delivery room by the obstetrician, during the neonatal examination by the pediatrician, or by the mother when changing diapers. The mass usually enlarges during crying spells. It is usually cystic, containing either clear or milky mucoid material. The differential diagnosis includes ecoptic ureter, hymeneal cyst, hymeneal skin tag, periurethral cyst, vaginal cyst, or imperforate hymen with hydrocolpos.

The child should be examined in the frog-leg position, ideally with

Clinical Practice of Gynecology: **3,** 146–160, 1989

magnification, using a moistened Q-Tip for retraction. The "pull-down" maneuver opens the introitus so that the origin of the cyst can be ascertained.

Ectopic Ureter

If the cyst appears to rise from the periurethral area or anterior vagina, ectopic ureter should be suspected and a pelvic and renal ultrasound obtained. If this diagnosis is confirmed, then consultation with a pediatric urologist is required. Usually, an intravenous pyelogram is obtained to determine the extent of the anomalous collecting system. High ligation of the ectopic ureter or partial nephrectomy is usually required.

Hymeneal, Periurethral, and Vaginal Cysts

Cysts arising from the hymen or periurethral area are usually of the epidermal inclusion variety. Spontaneous resolution is common. If regression does not occur within 3 months, then simple marsupialization or electrofulgeration is warranted. Before one proceeds with surgery, however, it is wise to examine the patient with a urethroscope to rule out the presence of a diverticulum of the distal urethra, which would require management by a urologist.

In the newborn period, vaginal cysts can be located posterior to the urethral meatus at the vaginal introitus arising from the anterior or lateral wall of the vagina and lined by squamous epithelium. Usually they do not cause pathologic manifestations and can rupture spontaneously, or they disappear after surgical aspiration and removal of a milky white fluid. Occasionally, the cysts grow large enough to obstruct the urethra, causing urinary retention. Operative removal is indicated in such cases. Cysts in the caudal portion of the vagina probably are derived from the epithelium of the urogenital sinus and formed during the last months of gestation. Multiple cysts can occur in proximal parts of the vagina. They have been considered derivatives of epithelia of the müllerian or Wolffian ducts.

Imperforate Hymen and Hydrocolpos

When the cystic structure appears to obstruct the vaginal opening, and no perforation can be identified, an imperforate hymen with hydrocolpos is the most likely diagnosis. In most cases, a hydrocolpos of varying size is also present. Hydrocolpos is due to distention of the vagina with retained secretions. The uterus is rarely involved because of the ability of the vagina to distend. The usual presenting symptoms of a massive hydrocolpos in the neonate are a midline lower abdominal mass, urinary retention caused by bladder angulation, and, on occasion, respiratory distress. Bilateral hydroureter and hydronephrosis may be detected on an antenatal ultrasound examination. Compression of the ureters at the pelvic brim may also be present.

Respiratory distress may result from pressure on the diaphragm. Lower extremity edema may be caused by compression of the major abdominal veins. We have seen one patient in whom retrograde flow of secretion through the fallopian tubes caused intraperitoneal adhesions and partial bowel obstruction.

The treatment of hydrocolpos depends upon its etiology. Surgery is indicated when it can avoid late complications of further fluid accumulation and reflux. Usually a simple hymenectomy, carried out in the nursery when the hydrocolpos is small, with a Beaver blade, is adequate. No bleeding occurs, and sutures are not required. In the older child, hymenotomy and drainage of the fluid should be managed in the ambulatory operating room under general anesthesia.

We have encountered three patients who presented with a unilateral cystic mass. When drainage was carried out, a vaginal septum with unilateral obstruction and hydrocolpos was diagnosed. This müllerian abnormality usually is associated with duplication of the cervix and uterus (didelphia), which can either be partial or complete. Since this anomally is frequently associated with urologic malformations, investigation of the ureters and kidneys should be undertaken. The same problem is not encountered with simple imperforate hymen.

Other Hymeneal Abnormalities

Hymeneal tags can be present at birth and appear as a fleshy mass protruding from the introitus. They frequently regress when the effects of maternal estrogen have diminished. If they are still present at 3 months, then they can be removed by electrocautery or cold knife excision, because if large enough, they become inflamed and cause vaginal bleeding and discharge.

Inadequate perforation of the hymen, such as septation, microperforation, or cribiform fenestration, is generally asymptomatic in the young child and does not require intervention until puberty, when it causes problems with tampon use and coitus. However, these separations should be operated upon when they appear to be the cause of recurrent vulvovaginitis and urinary tract infections caused by stagnation of urine within the partially obstructed vagina. Since most patients with this problem present between the ages of 3 and 6 years, either hymenectomy or hymenotomy and suturing the cut edges with absorbable sutures are satisfactory methods of treatment.

Inguinal Ovary

Inguinal hernias in female infants are generally uncommon with a male to female ratio of about six to one. When a 1.5-cm firm mass is palpated in the groin or vulva, it usually indicates that the hernia is of the sliding type where a portion of the wall of the sac is composed of a tube and ovary. It frequently cannot be reduced, but rarely the blood supply is compromised.

Rarely, a girl with a palpable gonad in the labia is actually a male with the testicular feminization syndrome. This represents less than 1% of hernias in females. These patients can also be identified by the findings of a 46XY karyotype and the operative findings of testicles. Early identification of these individuals is desirable, although there can be no gender changes made because the genitalia are female.

Cloacal Anomalies

A cloaca is a common channel into which the products of the gastrointestinal, urinary, and genital tracts empty. The pathogenesis of faulty cloacal division is unknown, but it could result from an arrest in the descent of the urorectal septum, preventing division of the cloaca into the rectum and urogenital sinus. This also stops approximation and fusion of the müllerian ducts, resulting in failure in the formation of the müllerian tubercle and a duplication of the uterus and proximal vagina. The sinovaginal bulbs do not form, and the vaginal plate does not enlarge. The urogenital sinus remains in its primitive state—a long, narrow tube—and the urethra empties into the urogenital sinus, high on its anterior wall. The hymen is absent.

A cloacal anomaly involves three major organ systems with the findings of complete or partial obstruction of the urinary, genital, or gastrointestinal tracts. In the absence of other lethal anomalies, urinary tract sepsis caused by obstruction accounts for the majority of deaths. The five major types of cloacal dysgenesis are as follows:

Type A has a single perineal orifice located between the labia minora. This orifice leads to a long, narrow tube—the cloaca—at the apex of which is an obstructed vagina. The urethral meatus enters the cloaca high on its anterior wall directly across from the posterior rectal fistula.

Type B is similar to Type A, but the rectal fistula enters the vagina. Type C has a short, broad cloaca. Type D is similar to Type A, but a distal vaginal atresia is present. Type E has a high type of imperforate anus but no rectocloacal fistula.

Other major system anomalies are common, particularly in the cardiovascular, genitourinary, gastrointestinal, central nervous, and respiratory systems. The most common anomalies are those of müllerian origin: septate vagina, duplication of the uterus, and bicornuate uterus.

The pathognomonic physical finding in cloacal dysgenesis is a single perineal orifice between the labia minora. This opening is the entrance to the cloaca. If the hymen is present, cloacal dysgenesis is not. The urethral meatus and anus are not evident. Hydrometrocolpos is often present as an abdominal mass. Reconstruction is complex and best performed by a pediatric surgeon.

Ambiguous Genitalia in the Newborn

Although most clinicians will rarely see an infant with ambiguous genitalia at birth, the need to assess the situation as quickly as possible makes this subject essential for inclusion in this chapter. Any deviation from the normal appearance of male or female genitalia should prompt investigation, since apparent, but incomplete, male or female external genitals may be associated with the gonads and genotype of the opposite sex (eg, the male with feminizing testicular syndrome, and the markedly virilized female with congenital adrenocortical hyperplasia [CAH]). Even a slight doubt that arises in the initial newborn examination should be pursued systematically to prevent the possibility of later confusion. Bilateral cryptorchidism, unilateral cryptorchidism with incomplete scrotal fusion or hypospadias, labial fusion, or clitoromegaly require evaluation.

DETERMINING SEX ASSIGNMENT

When the physician finds that an infant has ambiguous genitalia, the parents should be reassured that they have a healthy baby, but because the external genital development is incomplete, tests are necessary to determine the sex. A straightforward explanation of the factors necessary for normal sexual development in utero may be helpful. Clearly, most parents will react with dismay and anxiety; they should be reassured that tests will show the cause of the problem and whether their baby is a girl or a boy. The possibility of an intersex disorder (hermaphroditism) should not be raised at this time. Speculation about possible sex assignment should be kept to a minimum. Within a few days, or at most 1–2 weeks, a definite answer will be possible. The physician should examine the baby in the presence of the parents and explain the common genital anlage for boys and girls. The concept of an "underdeveloped" male or "overdeveloped" female helps parents accept their baby's condition.

Although a diagnosis of the patient's condition requires knowledge of the genotype, assignment of sex is based on other criteria as well. The first issue is fertility. The female with CAH may be virilized at birth, yet with normal ovaries and uterus, she is potentially capable of bearing children. Thus, management, including surgery, must aim at female gender identity. When fertility is not possible, as with mixed gonadal dysgenesis (MGD) or male pseudohermaphroditism, decisions are based on surgical requirements for reconstruction of the external genitals. In general, surgical techniques are more suited to clitoral recession and, later, the creation of a vagina, than to the construction of a normal male phallus. Once the decision as to sex assignment is made, the physician should help the parents accept their infant as a normal male or a normal female. As long as attitudes toward the child's sex remain unequivocal, the child usually assumes his or her gender role without difficulty, regardless of the genotype.

CONGENITAL ANOMALIES IN POSTPUBERTAL AGE GROUP

Labial Minora Hypertrophy or Asymmetry

In some instances, one or both labia minora are unusually large, and the patient consults because she notices the anomaly or because of symptoms of irritation associated with exercise. In most of these cases, simple reassurance is necessary. Comparison with asymmetry or hypertrophy of other parts of the body may help the patient to accept this peculiarity. Hygiene counseling and avoidance of right clothes are usually sufficient to relieve discomfort. When these measures prove to be ineffective, or in the presence of troublesome cosmetic problem, surgical reduction is in order. This can be accomplished in the ambulatory operating room by simply resecting the redundant labia so that they are symmetrical. Closure of the excised area is best accomplished with a running locking stitch of 3-0 chromic. The results are usually excellent, and the patients are generally quite pleased.

Congenital Adrenal Hyperplasia

In female pseudohermaphrodism caused by congenital adrenal hyperplasia, the external genitalia can be affected variously. The external urinary meatus is found most often at the base of the phallus, but sometimes it is extended to its end, where a glans penis and a prepuce are present, as in the male. There is a median perineal raphe, formed by scrotolabial folds in which no gonads can be felt. A vaginal opening is not always found externally, but cystoscopy reveals an opening on the floor of the urethra several centimeters from the vesical orifice representing the distal end of the vagina. The vaginal size and length differs. The common urethrovaginal canal opening onto the perineum represents a urogenital sinus. If prenatal virilization is less progressed, there are separate urethral and vaginal openings. Similar external genital changes may exist in female pseudohermaphrodites without adrenal disorders. Uterus, tubes, and ovaries are normally formed. The vagina may be absent in female pseudohermaphrodites who are masculinized by a maternal virilizing tumor or by androgens or progestins administered to the mother during pregnancy. The internal genitalia are female in such children, and there are no renal anomalies. The nature of the reconstructive surgery required varies with the anomaly but usually includes clitoral recession and perineoplasty with exteriorization of the vagina.

Imperforate Hymen with Hematocolpos (or Hydrocolpos)

Although the diagnosis of an imperforate hymen should be made long before adolescence, during routine neonatal and pediatric examinations, it is not infrequent to see a teenager present with the typical picture of primary amenorrhea, cyclic or acyclic pelvic pain, bulging hymen, and hematocolpos. Hematometra does not usually develop with simple imperforate hymen because the vagina has great distensibility and can accommodate a large amount of blood. However, it is quite commonly seen with high transverse septa.

Imperforate hymen can be congenital and due to failure of degeneration of central epithelial cells of the hymenal membrane; some cases may be the result of inflammatory processes before or after birth. If the vagina and the uterus are not distended by estrogen-induced secretions at the time of birth, the imperforate hymen may remain symptomless to the age of puberty, when collection of menstrual material results in enlargement of the vaginal tract, causing pelvic or abdominal pain.

Approximately two-thirds of the cases become manifest before the age of 15 years. A cystic mass is formed by enlargement of the vagina and uterus that can extend above the symphysis and into the abdominal cavity. Abdominal pain is a regular symptom, and urinary difficulties may develop. Many patients who are inadequately examined undergo extensive radiologic evaluation before the diagnosis is finally made. Examination of the external genitalia reveals a mass protruding between the labia majora. The bulging mass is variable in size, bluish red in color, and continuous with the pelvic mass. Constipation results in some cases because of pressure on the rectum from the distended vagina.

The surgical therapy consists of hymenotomy, which often reveals a large accumulation of blood or secretion. Excision of the central part of the hymen should also be carried out to allow further unobstructed menstrual flow. We have found that the utilization of needle-tip electrocautery facilitates hemostatis on the hymenal edge. This avoids the need for multiple sutures and minimizes the likelihood of secondary retraction. The use of a Yankauer suction tip inserted high into the vagina or through the dilated cervix into the uterus facilitates evacuation. At times, the wall suction becomes plugged, and a high-speed suctional evacuation is required. Infection is rare once drainage is established, and prophylactic antibody therapy is not required.

Microperforate, Cribriform, and Septate Hymen

Incomplete fenestration of the hymenal opening is most often asymptomatic. These patients seek gynecologic treatment because of unsuccessful attempts at inserting tampons or coital difficulties. With a microperforate hymen, the adolescent may also complain of postmenstrual vaginal spotting or malodorous discharge secondary to incomplete obstruction and poor drainage. Hymenectomy should be performed in all cases.

When the diagnosis is made fortuitously, the patient should be told about this anatomic variant and be informed of the necessity of surgical correction. Performing the procedure during the early teens allows the adolescent to use tampons without problems and may avoid later embarrassment when the patient desires to become sexually active.

Vaginal Agenesis

Vaginal agenesis in any of its forms is rare. There are three types: total agenesis (the Rokitansky–Kuster–Hauser syndrome), proximal atresia, and distal atresia. Only distal vaginal atresia results in hydrometrocolpos. Total vaginal agenesis results from failure of the müllerian ducts to reach the urogenital sinus. Other müllerian derivatives, the uterus and fallopian tubes, are frequently absent or represented only by rudimentary structures. Proximal vaginal atresia results from failure of fusion of the müllerian ducts at their tips so that the vaginal plate does not form. The cervix is absent, but the uterus and tubes are present. Distal vaginal atresia results from failure of the sinovaginal bulbs to proliferate. The proximal vagina, cervix, uterus, and tubes are intact. The urogenital sinus remains as a long, narrow tubular structure distal to the atresia, and, thus, the urethra is located within the urogenital sinus high on its anterior wall.

Vaginal agenesis is rarely diagnosed in the newborn girl. Usually it is identified after the expected time of menarche when menstruation does not occur. Since the ovaries are present, development of secondary sexual characteristics occurs. Cyclic pain and an abdominal mass are indicative of hematocolpos. Absence of menses and lack of cyclic pain indicate agenesis of both vagina and uterus.

Proximal vaginal atresia may present in the newborn period as an abdominal mass but most often is identified after the expected time of menarche because of cyclic abdominal pain, an abdominal mass, and lack of menstruation. Distal vaginal atresia most often presents in the newborn period with an abdominal mass caused by hydrometrocolpos. It may be a genetic disorder, inherited as a simple recessive trait.

In complete vaginal agenesis, the labia are underdeveloped, and there is a single opening between them. The normal vaginal introitus is absent. The patient with proximal vaginal atresia has a normal female perineum. The uterus is palpable on rectal examination. Vaginoscopy reveals a blind-ending vagina without a uterine cervix.

The pelvic examination of these patients reveals an absent vagina, and a particular feature is the small space separating the urethral meatus from the anus. The outer part of the vagina may be present as a blind vaginal canal of variable depth. This finding is more likely to be associated with testicular feminization syndrome. The presence or absence of a uterus is ascertained by rectoabdominal examination. External genitalia are usually of normal appearance. In cases of testicular feminization, characteristic stigmata can usually be observed.

The minimal workup should consist of pelvic ultrasound to confirm the presence or absence of a uterus, renal echography or intravenous pyelography to detect urinary tract anomalies found in approximately one-third of patients with müllerian agenesis, plasma testosterone level that will be in male range in case of testicular feminization syndrome, and a karyotype.

Plain roentgenograms of the chest, abdomen, and pelvis should be obtained first to identify associated pulmonary, cardiac, or bony anomalies. A urosonogram should be obtained in all patients with vaginal atresia. Injection of contrast media into any abnormal orifice also helps to clarify the complex anatomy.

Cystoscopy should be performed under anesthesia at the time of definitive treatment. The urethral meatus is found on the anterior wall of the urogenital sinus in the patient with distal atresia, but it is in the normal position in the patient having proximal vaginal atresia.

Associated anomalies are common in about one-third of the patients. Pelvic, kidneys, solitary kidneys, fused kidney, duplication of ureter or renal pelvis, and other anomalies are noted. Spina bifida, hemivertebrae, and irregularities of the ribs are occasional findings. Rarely, absence of the vagina is combined with normal internal genitalia, resulting in blockage of menstrual discharge, hematometra, and hematosalpinx. Amenorrhea is considered a manifestation of absence or deficiency of the uterus.

The important point is that this syndrome seems to be part of a complex of congenital malformations occurring in females with 46XX karyotype that include single kidney, bifid ureter, scoliosis, pectus excavatum, syndactyly, and situs inversus. It has long been known that renal anomalies are frequent in women with vaginal agenesis. Pelvic kidney, solitary kidney, horseshoe kidney, and ureteric and pelvic duplications had been observed. Every case of vaginal agenesis should be examined for renal anomalies.

Therapy of vaginal agenesis aims at the creation of a vaginal canal to allow satisfactory sexual function and to establish adequate menstrual drainage when a functioning uterus is present. Therapeutic management should be individualized for each patient.

When obstruction to menstrual flow is not a concern, therapy is best delayed until the patient desires the treatment done and has acquired enough maturity to comply with the demanding postoperative care that is the key to a successful outcome. In patients who already have a vaginal depth of 3 cm or more, treatment is not always needed, since coital activity may be sufficient to induce vaginal deepening. When a rudimentary vagina is present, the nonsurgical Frank method, which consists of progressive vaginal dilatation using dilators, should be attempted first.

The first attempt at vaginal reconstruction for vaginal agenesis was by Dupuytren in 1817. Since that time, numerous reports have appeared on vaginal reconstruction with the use of a multitude of materials, including intestine, both small and large, peritoneum, amniotic membrane, hernial sacs, and bladder, as well as nonsurgical stretching procedures.

The timing of vaginal reconstruction is important. In the newborn infant with vaginal atresia and hydrometrocolpos or cloacal dysgenesis, immediate separation of genital and urinary tracts is necessary, so vaginal reconstruction is a logical and desirable part of the operation. However, if there is total vaginal agenesis, reconstruction is easier and more satisfactory if done at maturity. Patients who are first diagnosed as having atresia at menarche should have their vaginas reconstructed at that time. There is no advantage in waiting until the patient is "ready" for sexual activity. In fact, the patient's self-image may be irreversibly damaged, should the situation be allowed to exist for a prolonged period once physical maturity has been reached.

The most commonly used technique in adolescents is that described by McIndoe, in which a neovagina is constructed by the use of split-thickness skin graft placed in a space created between the urethra and the rectum. A split-thickness skin graft (0.015–0.018 in.) is taken from the lower abdomen or buttocks and sutured in a spiral fashion to an acrylic or pliable silicone mold with absorbable sutures, so that the epidermis is in contact with the mold. With the use of a transverse incision, two parallel tunnels are created on either side of the urethra, deepened 8–12 cm, and united in the midline behind the urethra. Care must be taken to avoid entering either the urethra or the rectum. During the dissection, absolute hemostasis is mandatory. The epidermis-covered mold is then inserted into the tunnel, where it remains for 7–8 days. The patient is kept in bedrest for this period, and on the 8th day the mold is removed, the neovagina is cleansed, and the mold is reinserted. It is important that the mold be worn for at least 3 months postoperatively, until the contracture phase of the skin graft has ended. There are many modifications of this procedure.

Williams' vulvovaginoplasty is an acceptable therapeutic alternative. This technique offers the advantages of a shorter operative time, does not necessitate a skin graft, and has less risk of permanent stenosis if the patient does not comply with postoperative dilatation. Williams' procedure is most often performed to lengthen a preexisting rudimentary vagina or when the result of McIndoe's procedure is not satisfactory.

When a functioning uterus and cervix are present, treatment cannot be delayed because of obstruction to menstrual flow. In these cases, the principal problem is the young age at which surgical correction is necessary. Creation of a neovagina with the use of a centrally opened stent allowing drainage of menstrual blood that is left in place for 4–6 months decreases the likelihood of irreversible stenosis.

Vaginal Septa

A vaginal septum is a relatively uncommon anomaly. Septa can be either congenital or acquired, can occur in various positions, and can be multiple. Transverse septa can occur at any level from above the hymeneal ring to the junction of the vagina and cervix. Vertical septa can be oriented in an anteroposterior plan (sagittal septum) or in the lateral plane (coronal septum). Finally, septa can be complete or partial, perforate or imperforate.

Transverse vaginal septa occur from lack of complete canalization of the solid primitive vaginal plate or sinovaginal bulbs. Vertical vaginal septa occur in two ways. Failure of the müllerian ducts to fuse results in a duplication of the uterus and vagina. What appears to be a vertical vaginal septum is in fact a duplicated vagina. Two vaginal openings are found. In others, incomplete canalization of the vaginal plate in a longitudinal direction results in a septum that may be oriented in either the anteroposterior or the lateral plane. The symptoms produced by vaginal septa depend upon the age of the patient, the degree of vaginal obstruction, and the amount of stimulation of the cervical mucous glands by circulating estrogen. The neonate with a completely obstructed vagina caused by a transverse septum may present with hydrometrocolpos. However, a transverse vaginal septum may not be recognized until the patient reaches menarche, when hematocolpos develops. The neonate or older patient with a complete vertical septum may present with a unilateral hydrocolpos or hematocolpos, whereas an older patient with an incomplete vertical septum may seek help for dyspareunia or, if pregnant, for difficulty in delivery.

Symptoms depend on the width as well as the location of the anomaly. A narrow annular septum usually is a fortuitous finding of no clinical significance and does not require any treatment. On the other hand, primary amenorrhea and early symptoms of obstruction occur in cases of complete septum, and surgical excision is then imperative. When the upper and lower vagina communicates only by a small fistulous tract through the septum, the clinical picture is sometimes quite puzzling. These patients may present with dysmenorrhea, irregular vaginal spotting, or purulent discharge because of partial obstruction and accumulation of blood above the defect. Secondary pelvic inflammatory disease caused by anaerobic infection may also be the initial mode of presentation. A septum lying low in the vagina is frequently the cause of dyspareunia. Infertility and soft tissue dystocia are unusual presentations of this malformation in the adolescent group.

Surgical correction consists of complete excision of the septum and anstomosis of the upper vagina to the lower vagina. The utilization of a stent may be necessary when the septum involves a long vaginal segment and primary anastomosis is impossible. Care must be taken not to injure the urethra or rectum.

Postoperatively, periodic vaginal examinations at 6-week intervals should be performed with dilatations as necessary. Recurrence is rare if the septum is entirely excised. Postoperatively, stricture is rarely encountered. In some patients, however, the fallopian tubes will have developed some degree of fibrosis, because of pyocolpos with backflow prior to treatment.

Longitudinal vaginal septa most often occur in association with abnormalities of uterine fusion but may sometimes be an isolated malformation. Such septa divide the vagina sagittally in two equal or unequal parts for its entire length, or partially. Surgical excision is indicated when dyspareunia becomes a problem or when childbearing is anticipated.

In some instances, the septum fuses with the lateral vaginal wall and creates a blind vaginal pouch, giving rise to obstructive symptoms. This entity will be discussed together with obstructing uterine fusion anomalies.

Uterine Malformations

Uterine malformations can be divided into two main groups: 1) deficiencies (agenesis or degeneration), and 2) duplications. The relationship of these malformations to genic, chromosomal, or exogenous teratogenic factors is still not clear in most cases, although some progress has been made in etiologic classification.

CERVICAL AGENESIS

Congenital absence of the cervix can occur in association with vaginal agenesis or with a normal vagina. This rarity causes early obstructive signs and symptoms characterized by hematometra, tubal regurgitation or menstrual blood, and secondary endometriosis.

Attempts to preserve fertility by creation of a fistulous tract between the endometrial cavity and the vagina have been very disappointing. A conservative surgical approach usually leads to multiple repeated operations and even deaths. Only two successful pregnancies are reported in the literature. The recommended therapy of cervical agenesis, therefore, remains hysterectomy with ovarian conservation, when possible.

UTERINE AGENESIS

Absence of the uterus is noted in some apparently female patients who have the syndrome of male pseudohermaphrodism with testicular feminization. Such persons are genetic males, have negative sex chromatin and XY karyotype. They do not menstruate and cannot bear children, but their external genitalia are normal female, and they feminize at puberty, with good breast development. In rare cases, rudimentary tubes and uteri can be present. There are intraabdominal or inguinal testes with nests of Leydig cells.

The uterus is absent also in the majority of male pseudohermaphrodites with ambiguous genitalia. They may have testes situated intraabdominally, in the inguinal canal or in the scrotum. The vagina can be of differing size and length, often communicating with a hypospadic urethra. A minority of male pseudohermaphrodites with ambiguous external genitalia have a uterus and tubes. This can be of practical importance if, at laparotomy, gonads at the site of ovaries are seen in a child with tubes, uterus, and vagina. Such gonads can be testes.

UTERINE DUPLICATION WITH OBSTRUCTION

Abnormalities of uterovaginal fusion that are diagnosed during adolescent years are mostly those of the obstructing type. These anomalies can be divided into three categories according to the site of obstruction. Our experience at The Children's Hospital with 28 cases of uterine and/or vaginal obstructing duplications revealed that the most commonly encountered anomaly is a didelphic uterus with unilateral vaginal obstruction secondary to a blind vagina. Unicornuate uterus with a contralateral blind horn, either rudimentary or of normal size, is second in frequency. Finally, a small number of patients present with cervical obstruction of one horn of a bicornuate uterus associated with an ipsilateral blind vaginal pouch. Fistulous tracts of various types may connect the blind vagina to a septate cervix and/or to the main vaginal cavity. Intercervical fistula have also been discovered.

Signs and symptoms depend on the type of the abnormality. Since, in these cases, the obstruction is present only on one side, primary amenorrhea is not a feature. By far the most common presenting complaint is pelvic pain, either cyclic or acyclic, which is the consequence of unilaterally obstructed menstrual flow and secondary endometriosis. Other frequent symptoms include abnormal vaginal bleeding and purulent discharge usually associated with a fistulous tract connecting the obstructed to the unobstructed side. In the presence of a blind vagina, distention with menstrual blood may give rise to vaginal pain or the sensation of pressure. On physical examination, masses corresponding to distended pelvic structures, abnormal uterine shape, and discharge from possible fistulas can usually be visualized or palpated.

The minimal workup of these patients should include a combined pelvic and renal sonogram and an intravenous pyelogram. In our series, unilateral renal agenesis was found in 75% of the patients. Associated vesicoureteral reflux has also been reported. Laparoscopy and a hysterosalpingogram should also be performed in order to determine the exact nature of the anomaly.

Therapy aims to preserve the reproductive function. In the presence of a unilaterally blind double vagina, the only treatment needed is a vaginal septectomy. In cases of a blind uterine horn, the type of surgery depends on the size of the obstructed horn and consists of either unification metroplasty or hemihysterectomy. When one is dealing with combined cervical obstruction, blind vaginal pouch, and fistulous tracts, vaginal septectomy should be performed. Furthermore, because of the cervical obstruction, a unification procedure with complete removal of the cervical septum should also be carried out. Associated endometriosis should be treated adequately when necessary.

Gynecologic Abnormalities of Bladder Exstrophy

Fortunately, exstrophy of the urinary bladder is an uncommon anomaly. To the parents of such an afflicted newborn infant, the condition is distressing, frightening, and repulsive. The term *exstrophy* comes from two Greek words: The prefix *exo* means outside of, and the verb *strophe* means to twist or turn about. The distraught parents see this condition as a twisted, inside-out urinary bladder accompanied by abnormal genitalia.

Girls always have a bifid clitoris. Several series report a high incidence of myelomeningocele, which is of significance in terms of sphincter incontinence. The distance from umbilicus to anus is foreshortened. Often the umbilicus is just cephalad to the exstrophic bladder, and some are associated with an omphalocele. The anal aperture is often close to the vagina.

Characteristically, the girl with bladder exstrophy presents to the gynecologist following puberty because of abnormalities of the lower abdominal and vulvar area that result from her urologic reconstruction. Examination reveals scarring and deformity of the mons pubis, asymmetry of the labia, a bifid clitoris, and introital stenosis. The upper tract is usually normal. Bladder exstrophy is one of the conditions that also lead to congenital prolapse of the uterus, myelodysplasia and spinal bifida being the other two. From the psychologic standpoint, these patients are quite distraught because of their strange appearance and frequently shun their emerging female sexuality. Therefore, it is quite important to reassure them that total reconstruction can be accomplished.

We have performed a number of these operations in which a monsplasty, Williams' vulvovaginoplasty, and Manchester procedure are performed in a one-stage operation. The results are usually excellent, and full function is restored. Pregnancy can occur, but delivery should be abdominal.

REFERENCES

1. Cali RW, Pratt JH: Congenital absence of the vagina. Am J Obstet Gynecol 1968;100:752.
2. Capraro VJ, Dillon WP, Gallego MB: Microperforate hymen; a distinct clinical entity. Obstet Gynecol 1974;44:903.

3. Chisholm TC: Exstrophy of the urinary bladder. In: Holder TW, Ashcroft KW, eds. Pediatric surgery. Philadelphia: WB Saunders, 1980:738–751.
4. Counseller VS, Davis CE: Atresia of the vagina. Obstet Gynecol 1968;32:528.
5. Dewhurst CJ: Practical pediatric and adolescent gynecology. New York: Marcel Dekker, 1980.
6. Donahue PK, Hendren WH: Intersex abnormalities in the newborn infant. In: Holder TM, Ashcroft KW, eds. Pediatric surgery. Philadelphia: WB Saunders, 1980: 858–890.
7. Jirasek JE: Normal sex differentiation. In: Sciarra JJ, ed. Gynecology and obstetrics. Philadelphia: JB Lippincott, 1984(vol 5):770.
8. Jones HW Jr, Heller RH: Pediatric and adolescent gynecology. Baltimore: Williams & Wilkins, 1966.
9. Koff AK: Development of the vagina in the human fetus. Contrib Embryol 1933;24:59.
10. McIndoe A: Treatment of congenital absences and obliterative conditions of the vagina. Br J Plast Surg 1950;2:254.
11. Muckle CW: Developmental abnormalities of the female reproductive organs. In: Sciarra JJ, ed. Gynecology and obstetrics. Philadelphia: JB Lippincott, 1984(vol 1):4.
12. Rock JA: Surgical correction of uterovaginal anomalies. In: Sciarra JJ, ed. Gynecology and obstetrics. Philadelphia: JB Lippincott, 1984(vol 1):chap 70.

CHAPTER 14

Management of Ovarian Masses in Children and Adolescents

Odette Pinsonneault, MD and
Donald Peter Goldstein, MD

Over the past decade, gynecologists have been consulted more frequently over the problem of ovarian masses during childhood and adolescence. The true incidence of this condition has probably not changed but the increasing use of ultrasound by pediatricians and family practitioners has led to the detection of many functional cysts that were previously undetected. Even though masses are functional and require only reassurance and follow-up, it is imperative that true ovarian neoplasms receive immediate attention and therapy. Therefore, it is important that gynecologists feel comfortable in the evaluation of a child or teenager with an adnexal mass.

DIFFERENTIAL DIAGNOSIS

The differential diagnosis of ovarian masses includes enlargements of other reproductive structures as well as masses of extragenital origin. These topics are purposely omitted in this chapter.

All types of ovarian tumors seen in the adult can also be encountered in children and adolescents. The relative incidence of each entity is quite different, however. For example, because of the high incidence of anovulatory cycles, functional masses are much more frequent in the adolescent. Furthermore, in this age group, neoplastic tumors are more likely to be of germinal rather than of epithelial origin.

Fortunately, in children and adolescents, only one in ten ovarian tumors is malignant.[1] It is difficult to obtain accurate statistics regarding the frequency of functional cysts because most studies are based on surgical reviews. Since a large number of patients with functional ovarian enlargement

Clinical Practice of Gynecology: **3,** 161–166, 1989
© 1989 Elsevier Science Publishing Co., Inc.
655 Avenue of the Americas, New York, NY 10010

ISSN 1043-3198/89/$3.50

Table 14-1. Pathologic Diagnosis of 242 Ovarian Tumors Treated Surgically at Children's Hospital Medical Center (Boston): 1928–1982

	N (%)
Tumorlike enlargements	76 (31)
Primary ovarian tumors	166 (69)
Germ cell tumors	118 (71)
Mature teratoma	78
Immature teratoma	17
Endodermal sinus tumor	14
Dysgerminoma	8
Choriocarcinoma	1
Epithelial tumors	27 (16)
Serous	14
Mucinous	12
Mixed	1
Sex cord—stromal tumors	21 (13)
Granulosa	10
Sertoli-Leydig	7
Thecoma	2
Fibroma	1
Unclassified	1

Adapted from Lack and Goldstein: Primary ovarian tumors in childhood and adolescence. In: Current problems in obstetrics and gynecology, Vol. VII, Chicago: Year Book Medical Publishers, Inc., 1984.

are treated expectantly and never undergo surgery, they are not included in this published series.

In a recent publication, Lack and Goldstein[2] presented their experience with 242 children and adolescents operated on for ovarian masses. The results of this study are summarized in Table 14-1. Thirty-one percent of the patients were found to have a tumorlike condition, including follicle, corpus luteum, and simple and endometriotic cysts. Of their 166 cases of primary ovarian tumors, there were 118 (71%) germ cell tumors, of which 78 (66%) consisted of benign mature teratoma. Of 27 epithelial tumors, 85% were benign. Twenty-one (13%) of their patients had a sex cord-stromal tumor, which is generally considered as a low-grade malignancy. These results are comparable to other similar reports.[3–6]

SIGNS AND SYMPTOMS

A considerable number of ovarian tumors are asymptomatic and are discovered fortuitously during a routine pelvic examination. Since most young patients do not consult for periodic pelvic examination, ovarian masses are often picked up when they become large enough to cause symptoms or to be felt by abdominal palpation. Smaller ovarian enlargements are frequently incidental ultrasonographic findings at the time of an examination performed for unrelated symptoms, such as pain. This accounts for a large number of consultations for masses that prove to be physiologic.

Symptoms are usually related to the location and size of the mass or to mechanical accidents, such as rupture, torsion, or hemorrhage. In the young prepubertal girl, pain is abdominal because of the reduced pelvic capacity and the fairly high position of the ovaries. In the older patient, symptoms are more often pelvic. Bladder and ureteral compression may also be encountered with larger masses. Malignant tumors that infiltrate the surrounding tissues may induce bowel obstruction. In cases of mechanical accidents to the tumor, symptoms develop acutely and are usually characterized by severe pain and peritoneal signs, including nausea and vomiting. In hormone-producing tumors, precocious puberty, menstrual irregularities, or virilization may lead to the diagnosis.

On pelvic examination, the mass can usually be palpated by rectoabdominal examination with the patient in the lithotomy position. As mentioned previously, ovarian tumors in children are often intraabdominal rather than pelvic and should be considered in the differential diagnosis of abdominal masses. Other physical findings depend on the degree of invasion of the tumor and its hormonal activity.

DIAGNOSTIC WORKUP

Ultrasound is an invaluable tool in the diagnosis of ovarian masses. It provides information about the size and location and consistency of the tumor (ie, whether it is cystic, solid, or complex). Ultrasound is also useful to determine the presence of free peritoneal fluid and ascites. A flat plate of the abdomen reveals the presence of calcifications that suggest a diagnosis of dermoid cyst. However, this information can also be obtained by ultrasonography.

The remainder of the workup depends on the clinical picture. In the presence of a solid or hormonally active tumor, blood should be drawn for human chorionic gonadotropin (HCG), alpha-fetoprotein, CA-125, and estradiol. Follicle stimulating hormone (FSH) and luteinizing hormone (LH) levels may help to differentiate a true precocious puberty responsible for a functional cyst from an estrogen-secreting tumor inducing a pseudoprecocious puberty. When hirsutism or signs of virilization are present, a testosterone level should be obtained. When malignancy is suspected, a preoperative metastatic workup, including chest x-ray, brain, liver and bone scan, liver function tests, and computed tomography (CT) scan should be done.

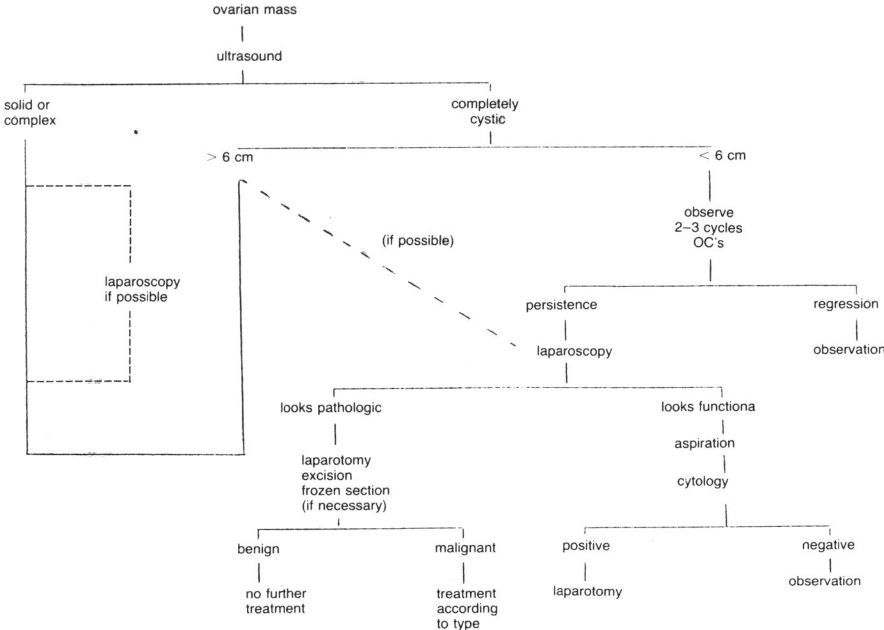

FIGURE 14-1 Management of ovarian tumors in the postmenstrual adolescent

MANAGEMENT

Postmenarchal Adolescent

In the postmenarchal patient, ovarian masses are approached quite similarly as in the young adult. Figure 14-1 summarizes the management of ovarian tumors in this age group. Upon the finding of an ovarian mass, ultrasound should be obtained to confirm the diagnosis and further define the tumor's characteristics. Because of the high incidence of functional masses, an asymptomatic, purely cystic tumor with a diameter of 6 cm or less is observed for 2–3 cycles for spontaneous regression. In these patients, the utilization of oral contraceptives to inhibit ovarian function may accelerate regression and prevent the appearance of new functional enlargement. Cystic masses that do not decrease in size over a period of 3 months, enlarge, or are larger than 6 cm initially should be operated on. A laparoscopy may be performed prior to laparotomy (when the size of the mass allows) in order to confirm the diagnosis. When the cyst appears to be functional and is less than 6 cm, puncture aspiration may be performed. All fluid obtained should be sent for cytologic examination.

Solid and complex tumors should be removed without delay. A laparoscopy may be performed as the initial procedure in order to establish the diagnosis and help decide on the optimal incision, and, in cases of unexpected malignancy, it allows the surgeon to discuss the extensiveness of the surgery with the parents.

Laparotomy should be performed through an incision large enough to allow excision of the tumor without rupture and according to the principles of ovarian surgery (ie, peritoneal lavage, complete abdominal exploration, frozen section, and periaortic node dissection when indicated). The surgical treatment of specific types of tumors is well described in the literature and will not be discussed in this chapter.

In cases of benign tumors, special care should be taken to preserve as much normal ovarian tissue as possible. Meticulous ovarian reconstruction should be carried out using microsurgical techniques in order to prevent adhesions and preserve reproductive function.

Premenarchal Child

In the premenarchal child, since the presence of a functional enlargement is unlikely, all ovarian tumors should be explored surgically. However, there are two exceptions to this rule. In the neonatal period, follicle cysts can develop because of the influence of maternal HCG or the withdrawal from high maternal estrogen and progesterone levels, which results in a transient secretion of gonadotropins by the newborn female. These cysts are usually of fairly large size. In 16 cases of follicle cysts in infants 6 months or younger reported by Lack and Goldstein,[2] the average diameter was 8.3 cm (3–16 cm). In these situations, the management depends on the size of the mass. When it is large enough to cause obstruction of the digestive or urinary tract, the cyst should be excised, in an attempt to preserve healthy ovarian tissue, if at all possible. Smaller cystic ovarian enlargements in the newborn can be observed for spontaneous regression, providing there is no evidence of torsion, hemorrhage, or rupture. The second period of childhood during which functional cysts may be encountered is the premenarchal period. In the premenarchal child, in whom sexual development has begun, an ovarian mass proved to be completely cystic by ultrasound can be safely managed according to the same criteria described for postmenarchal patients.

All solid or complex masses, no matter what the age of the patient, and cystic tumors occurring at any time of childhood except the neonatal and prepubertal periods, should be managed surgically.

REFERENCES

1. Barber HRK, Graber EA: Managing ovarian tumors in childhood and adolescence. Contemp Obstet Gynecol, 19;3:123–137.
2. Lack EE, Goldstein DP: Primary ovarian tumors in childhood and adolescence. In: Current

problems in obstetrics and gynecology, Vol. VII. Chicago: Year Book Medical Publishers, Inc., 1984.
3. Norris HJ, Jensen RD: Relative frequency of ovarian neoplasms in children and adolescents. Cancer 1972;30:713–719.
4. Abell MR, Holtz F: Ovarian neoplasms in childhood and adolescents, II Tumors of non-germ cell origin. Am J Obstet Gynecol 1965;93:850–866.
5. Moore JG, Schiffrin BS, Erez S: Ovarian tumors in infancy, childhood and adolescence. Am J Obstet Gynecol 1967;99:913–922.
6. Groeber WR: Ovarian tumors during infancy and childhood. Am J Obstet Gynecol 1963;86:1027–1035.

CHAPTER 15

Sterilization of the Unusual Adolescent Female

Odette Pinsonneault, MD and
Donald Peter Goldstein, MD

The need for sterilization of young nulliparous patients arises on rare occasions as an adjunct to the management of certain chronic conditions, such as cardiac, pulmonary and renal impairment, genetic diseases, and neuromuscular and severe seizure disorders. In these situations, contraception often becomes a problem because the choice is limited by numerous contraindications and patient compliance. Consequently, these patients may have to resort to less-than-optimal methods of birth control even though their needs may be as real as those of healthy teenagers. Therapeutic abortion is often not emotionally or morally acceptable for these young women and may be associated with increased morbidity because of their medical problem. Frequently, these young women develop tremendous anxiety regarding pregnancy because it could result in deterioration of their medical condition or in the birth of a baby that could be affected by a genetically transmitted disease or teratogenic medications. For these patients, the fear of bringing into the world a child for whom they feel unable to care for or whose risk of becoming orphaned prematurely is of great concern.

The decision to proceed to sterilization is never an easy one for the patient or for the physician. However, the situation must be faced realistically, particularly when the patient reaches emotional and physiologic maturity and tries to live as normally as possible despite her chronic illness.

This chapter presents experiences with tubal sterilization performed at The Children's Hospital (TCH), Boston, and analyses the different medical indications, techniques utilized, and complications encountered.

Clinical Practice of Gynecology: **3,** 167–170, 1989
© 1989 Elsevier Science Publishing Co., Inc.
655 Avenue of the Americas, New York, NY 10010

ISSN 1043-3198/89/$3.50

MATERIALS AND METHODS

Between June 1, 1977, and December 31, 1984, 27 patients ranging in age from 15 to 28 years of age underwent tubal ligation by laparoscopy at TCH. The hospital records were reviewed in order to obtain information on the age at the time of the procedure, the medical indications, the method of tubal sterilization, the type of anesthesia utilized, and the postoperative complications. Patients older than 19 years have been included purposely in this series even though they are beyond the adolescent group because it is the policy of our institution to continue to treat young adults who have been seen at TCH for a chronic disease since their childhood or adolescence. Furthermore, the sterilization procedure is often deliberately delayed until early adulthood in order to ensure that the patient is sufficiently mature and able to give informed consent.

RESULTS

The age at the time of sterilization ranged from 15 to 28 years with a mean of 21.8 years. Five patients were 19 years old or younger, while 22 were in their twenties. All procedures were performed on an inpatient basis when the primary disease was under optimal control. All tubal ligations were carried out by laparoscopy, 19 with Falope rings, 6 with Hulka clips, and 2 by electrocoagulation and division. General endotracheal anesthesia was utilized in 25 patients and local anesthesia in 2. The different clinical indications are summarized in Table 15-1.

There were two major postoperative complications encountered in two quite similar patients: Patient 1 was a 23-year-old black, single female with a past history of aortic and mitral valve replacement secondary to rheumatic disease treated with Coumadin and digoxin. After two therapeutic abortions, she decided to undergo a tubal ligation because she was not willing to run the risk of a full-term pregnancy. On admission, Coumadin was discontinued and intravenous heparin started. Heparin was stopped in the immediate preoperative period. Prothrombin time (PT) and partial thromboplastin time (PTT) were in optimal range at the time of surgery. She underwent an uneventful tubal ligation by laparoscopy using Falope rings. Coumadin was restarted approximately 12 hours after the procedure, and she was discharged on the second postoperative day without any evidence of bleeding. On the 8th postoperative day, she was readmitted with an acute abdomen. At laparotomy, 2 L of blood were found in the abdominal cavity. The source of the bleeding was from necrosis of the portion of the tubes occluded by the Falope rings. Bilateral salpingectomy was carried out. Two days later, a repeat laparotomy was performed because of recurrent intraabdominal bleeding. At this time, the bleeding originated at the site of

Table 15-1. Medical Indications for Tubal Sterilization in 27 Patients Aged 15–28 Years

	N
Pulmonary diseases	
Cystic fibrosis (mucoviscidosis)	11
Scoliosis with severely compromised respiratory capacity	1
Cardiac diseases	
Pulmonary hypertension	2
Status postvalve replacement under anticoagulation therapy	2
Pulmonary atresia and polycythemia	1
Tetralogy of Fallot and uncorrectable pulmonary atresia	1
Ebstein's disease with right to left shunt	1
Aortic stenosis (with Wilson's disease and severe mental retardation)	1
Renal diseases	
Renal insufficiency	1
Neurologic and neuromuscular diseases	
Severe seizure disorders	2
Seizure disorders and severe spastic hemiplegia	2
Friedreich's ataxia	1
Epilepsy (and systemic lupus erymatosus)	1

the cornual sutures. Hemostasis was finally accomplished, and the patient was discharged without any further complications.

Patient 2 was a 22-year-old white, single female with a past history of repair of an atrioventricular defect and mitral valve replacement. She was treated with Coumadin, digoxin, and Inderol. Her preoperative anticoagulation management was similar to that of patient 1. Because of the dramatic experience 3 years earlier with patient 1, it was elected to utilize Hulka clips to decrease the risk of hemorrhage caused by necrosis. Thirty-six hours postoperatively, she presented with signs of hemoperitoneum, which prompted a laparotomy. The source of the bleeding was from the infraumbilical laparoscope incision and from a small omental tear. No other surgical or anesthesia complications were encountered in the 25 other patients.

DISCUSSION

The whole issue of sterilization of young women represents an uncomfortable subject for the gynecologist as well as for the patient herself. Many different reasons may incite a young, chronically ill woman to ask for definite sterilization. When her medical condition poses an absolute contraindication to pregnancy, such as in primary pulmonary hypertension, or when the life expectancy is unfavorable, such as in cystic fibrosis or Friedreich's ataxia, the decision is usually less controversial. Most of the time, however, pregnancy is not absolutely contraindicated but carries the risk of compromising the mother's condition or of affecting the fetus. In these situations, the request of a mature young woman, who is not willing to run the risk or to comply with the physical restrictions of a high-risk pregnancy, should be respected. Consultation with the primary physician who has followed the patient for years and is well acquainted with her medical and emotional status is mandatory.

Even though the physician feels that sterilization is the optimal contraceptive modality, the patient should never be rushed into making this decision. In most instances, it is wise to have the patient seen by a psychiatrist or psychologist who can assist with the evaluation and provide subsequent emotional support, if required.

The procedure should be performed when the primary disease is under optimal control. The choice of the technique utilized depends on the gynecologist, who should opt for a method with which he or she feels comfortable and requires the shortest anesthesia time. When the patient is considered to be a good candidate for local anesthesia, this option should be considered, particularly if general anesthesia would be associated with a significant increase in morbidity.

The only two postoperative complications encountered in this series occurred in patients receiving anticoagulation therapy. On the basis of this experience, the safest technique would appear to be use of a Hulka clip applied at minilaparotomy.

CHAPTER 16

Gynecologic Problems in Adolescents with Chronic Diseases

S. Jean Emans, MD

Adolescents who have chronic diseases and malignancies that were fatal in the past have benefited from improved medical management and now seek care for a number of gynecologic problems. Even the healthy adolescent girl may have difficulties as she experiences pubertal changes and new sexual feelings; the adolescent with a chronic disease has special needs that must be understood and receive attention. Although this chapter will discuss only some of the common chronic diseases (cystic fibrosis, end-stage renal disease, diabetes mellitus, Crohn's disease, sickle cell disease, and malignancy), the physician needs to approach every adolescent with a sensitivity to her unique concerns. This sensitivity will enable the physician to treat patients with many other chronic diseases not mentioned in this chapter. Undoubtedly, an entire text could be devoted to the special gynecologic problems adolescents encounter in coping with a chronic illness.

CYSTIC FIBROSIS

Cystic fibrosis is the most common lethal hereditary disease in the white population. Although previously many children with cystic fibrosis died during infancy and early childhood, many patients with cystic fibrosis are living through their adolescence and into their reproductive years. Since these adolescents often have low weight for height and chronic pulmonary infections, they frequently experience a delay in pubertal development and menarchal age.[1-3] Neinstein[1] reported a delayed mean age of menarche for cystic fibrosis patients of 14.4 years compared to 12.9 years for U.S. females. Ninety-five percent of the postmenarchal patients weighed more than 82 lb, whereas 75% of amenorrheic adolescents weighed less than 82 lb. Ad-

Clinical Practice of Gynecology: **3,** 171–182, 1989
© 1989 Elsevier Science Publishing Co., Inc.
655 Avenue of the Americas, New York, NY 10010

ISSN 1043-3198/89/$3.50

olescents with delayed menarche were likely to be diagnosed with cystic fibrosis earlier in life, to have a lower weight for height index, a lower height, and a lower percent of body fat than postmenarchal girls. As a group, pubertal girls with cystic fibrosis have a mean estradiol level that is only 50% of the mean for age-matched controls.[3] Since normal levels of sex steroids and gonadotrophins are usually reached by most patients in their late teenage years, the adolescent with cystic fibrosis and amenorrhea should receive good medical and gynecologic assessment and supportive counseling. Other causes of amenorrhea, especially pregnancy, should be excluded, and reassurance should be given about the potential for normal menstruation.

The increasing use of ultrasonography has led to conflicting reports on the prevalence of ovarian cysts in patients with cystic fibrosis. Shawker and colleagues[4] reported that 46% of the ultrasounds in 13 menstruating women ages 13–38 years revealed ovarian cysts more than 3 cm in size. These cysts were unilateral, unilocular, and, in the few patients followed longitudinally, transitory. The overall incidence of cysts on the total of 16 ultrasound exams was 37.5%, compared to 7% among normal subjects. In contrast, Wang and colleagues[5] found only one ovarian cyst among 18 adults with cystic fibrosis but did note enlarged ovaries in 4 of the patients. Autopsy data on ovaries has not been conclusive. Shawker and colleagues[4] reported that none of the pathology specimens of 23 patients with cystic fibrosis had frank cysts greater than 2 cm in diameter. Cystic fibrosis patients had fewer grossly detectable follicles than did a control cardiac population, perhaps because the terminal illness in cystic fibrosis is frequently prolonged and may impair normal ovulation for a long duration prior to death.

The unusual characteristics of cervical mucus in patients with cystic fibrosis was recognized by Kopito and colleagues,[6] who reported the finding of thick tenacious cervical mucus that contained only one-quarter to one-third as much water as control mucus. The water content did not increase at midcycle, and a ferning pattern was not observed in any of the patients. The cervix may be chronically inflamed or have a pseudopolypoid ectropion.[7] The increased friability of the large ectropion may be particularly evident in patients who are taking oral contraceptives. Although some of the diminished fertility of cystic fibrosis patients has been attributed to this abnormally viscous cervical mucus that may provide a barrier to sperm penetration, pregnancies occur with sufficient frequency that it is mandatory for the adolescent with cystic fibrosis to receive contraceptive care.

The contraceptive choices for the patient with cystic fibrosis are not simple. Although the use of oral contraceptives does not appear to alter pulmonary function, long-term safety data is not available. The risk of fluid retention and other side effects with high estrogen pills necessitates the prescription of a low-dose pill. Weight, pulmonary and cardiac status, and liver function should be carefully monitored. Patients with preexisting chronic liver disease need careful assessment of the potential risks of pregnancy versus the unknown risk for potential hepatic effects. For most adolescents with cystic fibrosis, oral contraceptives are well tolerated and offer the many advantages of reliable contraception, diminished menstrual flow, and improved dysmenorrhea. Barrier forms of contraception can be used by the mature adolescent. An intrauterine device (IUD) is not recommended for most nulliparous adolescents and may be especially difficult to monitor in those adolescents with recurrent abdominal pain and severe constipation. Tubal ligation is an option for the young adult with cystic fibrosis who has made a definitive choice to avoid pregnancy.

In the last decade, many pregnancies have occurred in young women with cystic fibrosis.[8–12] The largest survey, by Cohen and di Sant'Agnese,[9] obtained data from 119 cystic fibrosis centers and provided information on 129 pregnancies in 100 patients. Thirty-one of these pregnancies were terminated by abortion (6 spontaneous and 25 therapeutic abortions), and 97 pregnancies were completed with 86 resulting in viable infants. The mean age of these young women was 20.7 years with a range of 17–34 years. Cystic fibrosis had been diagnosed at a mean age of 11 years. Since the mean age of diagnosis of cystic fibrosis in these centers was 3.7 years, a later age of diagnosis suggests milder disease in many of these patients. Unfortunately, 27% delivered at less than 37 weeks of gestation, and 11 perinatal deaths occurred. Maternal weight gain was less than 4.5 kg in 41% of cystic fibrosis patients versus 7% of controls. Adequate weight gain correlated with full-term births, whereas insufficient weight gain correlated with premature birth and stillbirth. The chance of a perinatal death was markedly increased by a history of dyspnea and cyanosis in the mother. The 15 women who died within 6 months postpartum had moderately severe to severe pulmonary disease with increasing symptoms during pregnancy.

The consensus of case reports and series of pregnant women with cystic fibrosis is that careful medical assessment is very important before a patient undertakes a planned pregnancy. Clinical criteria should optimally include the Shwachman–Kulczycki score, weight for height index, Brasfield chest radiograph score, and pulmonary function tests. Palmer and colleagues[11] found that the mother's overall condition after pregnancy tended to return to her pregravid level if her Shwachman–Kulczycki clinical score was over 74 and her weight for height was over 88%. Patients who did well with a pregnancy had near-normal Brasfield chest roentgenogram scores and had only mild to moderate airway obstruction and normal lung volume on pulmonary function tests. Women with low Shwachman–Kulczycki scores, poor nutrition, moderately to severely abnormal findings on chest x-rays, and restrictive-obstructive lung disease experienced pulmonary deterioration during their pregnancies, delivered premature infants, and did not return to their pregravidic health status postpartum.

On a few occasions, patients have been diagnosed with cystic fibrosis during a pregnancy because of recurrent respiratory symptoms, abnormal chest x-ray findings, abnormal pulmonary function tests, or hypoxia.[12] A woman with cystic fibrosis has approximately a 1 in 40 chance of having an infant with cystic fibrosis if the carrier status of the father is unknown (a 50% chance if the father is a heterozygote).[8] The clinician caring for the adolescent or young adult woman with cystic fibrosis needs to be sensitive to the issues confronting her: the genetic basis of the disease, her clinical status, and her prognosis.

CHRONIC RENAL DISEASE

Like many patients with other severe chronic diseases, adolescents with end-stage renal disease usually experience a delay in pubertal growth and development and menarche. Postmenarchal uremic patients on chronic dialysis rarely have regular menses.[13–18] For example, in a survey of 17 premenopausal patients, only 1 had regular menses, 6 had irregular menses with occasional spotting to dysfunctional uterine bleeding, and 10 were amenorrheic.[17] Hormonal studies revealed that the follicle stimulating hormone (FSH) levels were comparable to the levels of normal women (13.4 ± 1.5 mIU/mL in the uremic patients versus 15.0 ± 1.0 mIU/mL in control patients in the follicular phase). Luteinizing hormone (LH) levels were normal or increased (LH 18.6 ± 1.5 mIU/ml versus 10.9 ± 1.0 mIU/mL in normal women) and showed an absence of cyclicity. Administration of ethinyl estradiol (given for 4 days in the follicular phase) resulted in an increase in LH in normal women but not in uremic women.

Prolactin levels are often elevated in uremic patients on hemodialysis. Lim and colleagues[17] reported prolactin levels of 41.4 ± 5.8 ng/mL in uremic women versus 11.7 ± 1.1 ng/mL in controls; 7 of 17 women had galactorrhea. Hyperprolactinemia appears to be a direct consequence of impaired renal function.[17,18] Administration of bromocriptine to three patients led to resumption of menstruation in only one.[17] Associated with the chronic anovulation of uremia, two studies have suggested that ovarian cysts occur more commonly in patients on dialysis than in normal women.[19,20] Ovarian cysts may be asymptomatic or cause acute symptoms because of torsion or hemorrhage into the cyst (perhaps related to anticoagulant therapy). These ovarian cysts usually respond to hormone suppression therapy or resolve promptly after successful transplantation.

Uremic patients on dialysis usually require no therapy for the amenorrhea other than gynecologic assessment to exclude other etiologies for the amenorrhea. Although rare, pregnancy can occur in adolescents on dialysis. Two pregnancies were reported by Tegani and associates,[21] and one occurred at our medical center in a 15-year-old patient. Adolescents with dysfunctional uterine bleeding require assessment and, depending on the individual, treatment with oral progestins, oral contraceptives, and, if persistent, dilation and curettage (D & C).

Retrograde menstruation can occur in uremic patients as in normal women. Blumenkrantz and colleagues[22] observed that blood was regularly noted in the peritoneal dialysis catheter just before menstruation in 9 of 11 premenopausal patients who were having menses.

It is extraordinarily important for the adolescent who has had a successful renal transplant to understand that ovulation usually returns within 1–12 months after renal function approaches normal.[14,17,23,24] Adolescents may not appreciate the increase in fertility and may become pregnant post-transplant because of risk-taking behavior. Contraceptive counseling is paramount. If the adolescent has no contraindications (eg, hypertension) to the use of oral contraceptive pills, a low-dose formulation can be utilized. The IUD is not a good choice for the immunosuppressed nulliparous adolescent because of the potential for sepsis. Zerner and colleagues[23] have suggested that the pregnancy rate of the IUD may be increased because immunosuppressant agents impair the antifertility effect of the IUD. Barrier contraception is an acceptable option for the mature adolescent. By 1981, 440 pregnancies had been reported in transplant patients with a 70% successful outcome of those carrying to term.[23] Experience has continued to accumulate on pregnancy in transplant patients and the potential complications that include preeclampsia and prematurity.[25–29] Patients should have good renal status for a minimum of 2 years after a transplant before undertaking a pregnancy.

DIABETES MELLITUS

Adolescents with diabetes mellitus are more likely to experience a normal age for menarche than adolescents with other chronic illnesses. In a recent survey, Schriock and associates[30] found that adolescents with the onset of diabetes before age 11 years had menarche at a mean 13.1 ± 1.2 years (control nondiabetic population 13.0 ± 1.2 years), whereas adolescents with the onset of diabetes after 11 years had a delayed mean menarchal age of 14.0 ± 1.2 years. Postmenarchal adolescent diabetics may have irregular menses, dysfunctional uterine bleeding, and/or prolonged amenorrhea. Gonadotrophin and prolactin levels in amenorrheic diabetics are usually in the low to normal range despite low estradiol levels, suggesting depression of the hypothalamic–pituitary axis. Djursing and colleagues[31,32] have hypothesized that increased central/peripheral dopamine and/or cortisol activity in these patients may influence the hypothalamic–pituitary axis and result in amenorrhea.

Diabetic adolescents are often troubled by recurrent and persistent monilial vulvovaginitis. Improved diabetic control and the use of long-term antifungal vaginal medications can be quite helpful. Surprisingly, some diabetics who have marked swelling and erythema of the vulva in association with chronic candidiasis complain of little or no symptoms. Condyloma acuminata can also be a persistent problem, especially in poorly controlled diabetics with monilial vaginitis. Treatment with podophyllin therapy may result in suboptimal results. Since some diabetics develop extreme burning and irritation with podophyllin, the initial application should be limited to only a few warts, and the medication should be washed off within 1–2 hours. Other diabetic patients may have warts that are quite resistant to podophyllin and require a combination of improved glucose control, anti-monilial vaginal medications, and other forms of treatment.

Providing contraceptive services to diabetic adolescents involves balancing risks and benefits of each form of birth control. Oral contraceptives can alter glucose tolerance and lipoprotein levels and have been associated with increased vascular complications in diabetics.[33–36] Although optimally oral contraceptives should be avoided in diabetics, barrier forms of contraception may not be acceptable to the young risk-taking adolescent. Combined oral contraceptives such as ethinyl estradiol and lynestrenol appear to influence diabetic control slightly more than low-dose progestins.[33,34] Rådberg[33] has suggested that insulin-dependent diabetics appear to be more sensitive to the influence of 19-norprogestins than to alkylated estrogens with respect to lipid metabolism. Oral contraceptives do not appear to be associated with proliferative retinopathy, but the potential for accelerating the progression of this disorder remains a concern.[36] Thus, low-dose oral contraceptives with 30–35 µg of ethinyl estradiol and a low-dose progestin with minimal impact on glucose tolerance can be considered for adolescent diabetics, but medical status, blood glucose, and serum lipids should be monitored. Adolescents should be counseled to avoid smoking.

Although the complications of pregnancy in diabetics are well described and beyond the scope of this chapter, recent studies have suggested that excellent blood glucose control with near normal hemoglobin A_1C prior to conception can significantly reduce the incidence of congenital anomalies.[37–39] Counseling of adolescents should emphasize the long-term benefits of glucose control. A young patient should be enrolled in a high-risk program months before undertaking a planned pregnancy.

CROHN'S DISEASE

Adolescents with Crohn's disease may experience growth failure, pubertal delay, and menarchal delay. In fact, delayed growth may be the first manifestation of Crohn's disease and may not initially be recognized as secondary to a gastrointestinal problem. Gonadotrophins and estrogen levels are low and imply a depressed hypothalamic–pituitary axis. Nutritional and medical therapy, and sometimes surgery, to treat active Crohn's disease are important to assure normal pubertal growth and development. Although excess corticosteroids may impair growth, a patient with active Crohn's disease who receives doses that adequately treat the illness often has a growth spurt.

Adolescents with Crohn's disease may experience vulvar and perianal symptoms. Perianal lesions may be the first sign of the diagnosis of Crohn's disease. Characteristic vulvar lesions include edema of the labia majora and ulcerations in which skin granulomas are separated from the affected gastrointestinal (GI) tract by normal skin.[40] These ulcerations, which may resemble small herpetic lesions, last for weeks to months. Following proctocolectomy for Crohn's disease, some patients develop vaginal fistulas. A sinus tract may discharge onto the posterior wall of the vagina or directly onto the perineum. These fistulas have responded to long-term metronidazole therapy or surgery.

Because of the treatment with corticosteroids and immunosuppressive drugs, young women with Crohn's disease may experience recurrent monilial vulvovaginitis and condyloma acuminata. Adolescents can usually take oral contraceptives without difficulty, although a possible association between the prior use of oral contraceptives and "Crohn's disease" of the colon (but not ulcerative colitis) has been suggested.[41] A small number of cases of colitis associated with rectal sparing and segmental disease but *not* granulomas have been attributed to the use of oral contraceptives and have improved after oral contraceptives were stopped.[41] Thus, if a patient develops colitis during oral contraceptive use, the pills should be stopped to see if a remission occurs. Patients with true Crohn's disease associated with granulomas on colonic biopsy would not be expected to improve with cessation of oral contraceptives.

Many questions are unanswered in understanding the relationship of Crohn's disease to fertility and pregnancy. Two recent literature surveys have indicated the inadequacies of the studies in women with Crohn's disease: The health status of the patient and the severity of disease is often not defined, the husband is not evaluated, and the actual desire for fertility and the time of follow-up are not included.[42,43] Although many women with Crohn's disease do conceive and carry normal pregnancies, active Crohn's disease does appear to be associated with an increased risk of infertility. The "subfertility" may be related to the activity of a chronic disease, including malnutrition, perineal complications, and fistulas that may prevent normal coitus, and the deleterious effect of a pelvic abscess on Fallopian tube function. Crohn's disease does not appear to have an adverse effect on the fetus, although patients who have the onset of Crohn's disease during pregnancy or have active disease early in pregnancy appear to have a higher rate of spontaneous abortion.[43] Patients experiencing severe complications, such as an abscess or a bowel obstruction requiring surgery during pregnancy, also have an increased chance of adverse effects on their pregnancy. Sulfasalazine and corticosteroids are usually well tolerated during pregnancy, and pregnancy itself appears to have little effect on the course of the Crohn's disease. It has been estimated that 15–40% of patients with Crohn's disease will have an exacerbation during their pregnancy, and about an equal number will remain unchanged or improved.[43] The absence of problems with one pregnancy does not give an indication for the outcome of subsequent pregnancies. Postpartum recurrences of Crohn's disease can occur but may not be more frequent than the natural history of the disease. Since adolescents frequently have many questions about their ability to conceive and carry a pregnancy, it is important for the gynecologist to be knowledgeable about current data. The adolescent patient benefits greatly from hearing the optimism that pervades the current reviews on the potential for normal fertility and pregnancy.

SICKLE CELL DISEASE

Adolescents with sickle cell (SC) disease often have a delay in growth and development and a later age of menarche than their peer group. In a study of 96 children, Mann[44] found that the growth of children with SC disease was impaired in comparison to black children with sickle thalassemia or SC disease. A lean body habitus was more common among children with SS disease. The age of menarche for SS disease was 15 years versus 11.6 years for SC disease and 11 years for sickle thalassemia. In a sample of 91 Jamaican women with SC disease more than 15 years of age (range 15–65 years), Alleyn et al[45] reported a mean age of menarche of 15.4 ± 1.7 years compared to a control population of 13.1 ± 1.7 years. Longitudinal growth data in adolescent boys and girls with SS disease have shown a later age of the growth spurt when compared with the standards of Tanner.[46] The most comprehensive attempt to define growth data in children with hemoglobinopathies was reported by Platt and colleagues.[47] In a study involving over 2,000 patients with SS disease, SC disease, sickle β^+ thalassemia and sickle β° thalassemia, patients with SS and $S\beta^\circ$ were shorter on cross-sectional growth data than those with SC and $S\beta^+$. The weight curves followed a similar but more pronounced pattern than the heights; SS and $S\beta^\circ$ patients weighed less than SC and $S\beta^+$ patients. Analysis of Tanner staging showed that patients with SS and $S\beta^\circ$ were less mature than those with $S\beta^+$ and SC disease. When age and weight were included in the statistical model, menarchal status did not differ among the various hemoglobinopathies. Although SS and $S\beta^\circ$ patients experienced a clear delay in growth and development, the progression through the Tanner stages was normal. Platt concluded that the delay represented a constitutional delay and was not the result of a permanent gonadal or pituitary problem. The etiology of the low weight in SS and $S\beta^\circ$ remains unexplained, but Platt has suggested that the acute and chronic vasoocclusive crises may lead to poor nutritional intake. Patients with the more striking hemolysis that accompanies SS and $S\beta^\circ$ disease may have lower hematocrits, more marrow and cardiovascular compensation, and larger caloric requirements.

Adolescents with hemoglobinopathies require contraceptive counseling. Because of the concern for potential thromboembolic phenomenon in patients with vasoocclusive crises that include nephropathies and strokes, combined oral contraceptives are best avoided until more data can be gathered as to the benefits and risks of estrogen-containing pills. Although the risks of the minipill are unknown, they appear to be well tolerated. Other contraceptive choices include barrier contraception and for some patients, the IUD.

Pregnancies have been reported in many patients with SS disease. Perhaps because of delayed maturation and menarche, patients with SS disease may have pregnancies later than their normal peers.[45] In Alleyne's study, fetal wastage (miscarriages and stillbirths) was more common in patients with SS disease (22/112 [19.7%]) than normal patients (161/1699 [9.5%]). The first case of a successful pregnancy with SS disease and renal transplantation was reported in 1984.[48]

CHILDHOOD MALIGNANCY

With the survival into adulthood of many children, who previously would have died of malignancies, it is important for physicians to be aware of the gynecologic problems that occur among these patients. Chemotherapy for leukemia appears to have a minimal impact on later pubertal development and menses in girls in whom the diagnosis of leukemia was made before puberty began.[49] In contrast, girls who are diagnosed with leukemia and treated with chemotherapy after the onset of puberty or menarche may experience a delay in menarche and/or 2° amenorrhea. In almost all cases, menses eventually become normal.

Radiation therapy for solid tumors and lymphomas frequently results in permanent ovarian damage and ovarian failure. Data on long-term survivors of childhood malignancy found that ovarian failure occurred in 68% of patients who had both ovaries within abdominal radiotherapy fields, in 14% whose ovaries were at the edge of treatment fields, and in none of the patients with one or both ovaries outside an abdominal treatment field.[50] Adolescents with impaired ovarian function may experience either no adolescent sexual development or some estrogen effect at the normal pubertal age accompanied by primary or secondary amenorrhea. Gonadotrophin levels are elevated in the menopausal range, and estradiol levels are usually less than 30 pg/mL. Replacement therapy with estrogen and medroxyprogesterone can provide normal sexual development and, in most cases, menses. Some adolescents also develop vaginal adhesions that require dilators and hormonal therapy. Counseling should focus on the potential for normal development and sexual functioning. Medical follow-up should include routine examination, Papanicolaou smears, and bone densitometry. Patients should be instructed in adequate dietary calcium intake.

Acute gynecologic problems, such as dysfunctional uterine bleeding, may occur in the postmenarchal adolescent with leukemia and low platelets. The adolescent should be examined gently; ultrasonography may be helpful to exclude pelvic pathology if adequate bimanual examination is difficult in the virginal girl. Hormonal therapy, such as continuous low-dose birth control pills, can be prescribed to induce amenorrhea and endometrial atrophy until the patient has normal platelet function and can cope with normal menses.

Although many other chronic diseases are a problem for adolescents and have special consequences for the gynecologist who is following that patient, this chapter has dealt with some of the more common diagnoses. Hopefully, the specific issues described will make physicians conscious of the need to counsel adolescents and to provide medical treatment appropriate for adolescents' unique problems.

REFERENCES

1. Neinstein LS, Stewart D, Wang C, et al: Menstrual dysfunction in cystic fibrosis. J Adolesc Health Care 1983;4:153–157.
2. Moshang T, Holsclaw DS: Menarchal determinants in cystic fibrosis. Am J Dis Child 1980;134:1139–1142.
3. Reiter ED, Stern RL, Root AW: The reproductive endocrine system in cystic fibrosis; I. basal gonadotrophins and sex steroid levels. Am J Dis Child 1981;135:422–426.
4. Shawker TH, Hubbard VS, Reichert CM, et al: Cystic ovaries in cystic fibrosis: An ultrasound and autopsy study. J Ultrasound Med 1983;2:439–444.
5. Wang CI, Reid BS, Miller JH, et al: Multiple ovarian cysts in female patients with cystic fibrosis. Cystic Fibrosis Club Abstracts. Rockville, MD: Cystic Fibrosis Foundation. 1981:77.
6. Kopito LE, Losasky HJ, Shwachman H: Water and electrolytes in cervical mucus from patients with cystic fibrosis. Fertil Steril 1973;24:512–516.
7. Dooley RR, Braunstein H, Osher AB: Polypoid cervicitis in cystic fibrosis patients receiving oral contraceptives. Am J Obstet Gynecol 1974;118:971–974.
8. diSant'Agnese PA, Davis DB: Cystic fibrosis in adults. Am J Med 1979;66:121–132.
9. Cohen LF, di Sant'Agnese PA, Friedlander J: Cystic fibrosis and pregnancy: a national survey. Lancet 1980;2:842–844.
10. Corkey CW, Newth CJ, Corey M, et al: Pregnancy in cystic fibrosis: a better prognosis in patients with pancreatic function? Am J Obstet Gynecol 1981;140:737–742.
11. Palmer J, Dillon-Baker C, Tecklin JS, et al: Pregnancy in patients with cystic fibrosis. Ann Int Med 1983;99:596–600.
12. Johnson SR, Varner MW, Yates SJ: Diagnosis of cystic fibrosis during pregnancy. Obstet Gynecol 1983;61:25–75.
13. Swamy AP, Woolf PD, Cestero RV: Hypothalamic–pituitary–ovarian axis in uremic women. J Lab Clin Med 1979;93:1066–1072.
14. Morley JE, Distiller LA, Epstein S, et al: Menstrual disturbance in chronic renal failure. Horm Metab Res 1979;11:68–72.
15. Wass VJ, Wass JA, Rees L, et al: Sex hormone changes underlying menstrual disturbances on haemodialysis. Proc Eur Dial Transplant Assoc Eur Ren Assoc 1978;15:178–186.
16. Perez RJ, Lipner H, Abdulla N, et al: Menstrual dysfunction of patients undergoing chronic hemodialysis. Obstet Gynecol 1978;51:552–555.

17. Lim VS, Henriquez C, Sievertson G, et al: Ovarian function in chronic renal failure: evidence suggesting hypothalamic anovulation. Ann Intern Med 1980;93:21–27.
18. Gomez F, de la Cueva R, Wauters JP, et al: Endocrine abnormalities in patients undergoing longterm hemodialysis. The role of prolactin. Am J Med 1980;68:522–530.
19. Thaysen JH, Olgaard K, Jensen HG: Ovarian cysts in women in chronic intermittent haemodialysis. Acta Med Scand 1975;197:433–437.
20. Vaughan R, Henderson SC, Rahatzad M, et al: Unsuspected adnexal masses in renal transplant recipients. J Urol 1982;128:1017–1019.
21. Tejani A, Gurumurthy K, Sen D: Accidental pregnancies in teenage children on dialysis. NY State J Med 1982;82:1234–1235.
22. Blumenkrantz MJ, Gallagher N, Bashore RA, et al: Retrograde menstruation in women undergoing chronic peritoneal dialysis. Obstet Gynecol 1981;57:667–670.
23. Zerner J, Doil KL, Drewry J, et al: Intrauterine contraceptive device failures in renal transplant patients. J Reprod Med 1981;26:99–102.
24. Bierman M, Nolan GH: Menstrual function and renal transplantation. Obstet Gynecol 1977;49:86–89.
25. Fine RN: Pregnancy in renal allograft recipients. Am J Nephrol 1982;2:117–122.
26. Conlam CB, Zincke H, Sterioff S: Relationship between donor age and outcome of pregnancy in a renal allograft population. Transplantation 1982;33:97–99.
27. Rudolph JE, Schweizer RT, Bartus SA: Pregnancy in renal transplant patients: A review. Transplantation 1979;27:20–29.
28. Papoff P, Whetham JC, Katz A, et al: Pregnancy in renal transplant recipients: report of two successful pregnancies in a patient with impaired renal function. Can Med Assoc J 1977;117:1288–1295.
29. Whetham JC, Cardella C, Harding M: Effect of pregnancy on graft function and graft survival in renal cadaver transplant patients. Am J Obstet Gynecol 1983;145:193–197.
30. Schriock EA, Winter RJ, Traisman HS: Diabetes mellitus and its effect on menarche. J Adolesc Health Care 1984;5:101–104.
31. Djursing H, Nyholm HC, Hagen C, et al: Depressed prolactin levels in diabetic women with anovulation. Acta Obstet Gynecol Scand 1982;61:403–406.
32. Djursing H, Nyholm HC, Hagen C, et al: Clinical and hormonal characteristics in women with anovulation and insulin-treated diabetes mellitus. Am J Obstet Gynecol 1982;143:876–882.
33. Rådberg T, Gustafson A, Skryten A, et al: Oral contraception in diabetic women. Horm Metab Res 1982;14:61–65.
34. Rådberg T, Gustafson A, Skryten T, et al: Oral contraception in diabetic women. Diabetes control, serum and high density lipoprotein lipids during low-dose progestogen, combined oestrogen/progestogen and non-hormonal contraception. Acta Endocrinol (Copenh) 1981;98:246–251.
35. Steel JM, Duncan LJ: Contraception for the insulin-dependent diabetic woman: The view from one clinic. Diabetes Care 1980;3:557–560.
36. Steel JM, Duncan LJ: Serious complications of oral contraception in insulin-dependent diabetes. Contraception 1978;17:291–295.
37. Steel JM, Johnstone FD, Smith AF, et al: Five years' experience of a "prepregnancy" clinic for insulin dependent diabetics. Br Med J 1982;285:353–356.
38. Ylinen K, Raivo K, Teramo C: Haemoglobin A_1C predicts the perinatal outcome in insulin dependent diabetic pregnancies. Br J Obstet Gynecol 1981;81:961–967.
39. Miller E, Hare JW, Cloherty JP, et al: Elevated maternal hemoglobin A_1C in early pregnancy and major congenital anomalies in infants of diabetic mothers. N Engl J Med 1981;304:1331–1334.
40. Kremer M, Nussenson E, Steinfeld M, et al: Crohn's disease of the vulva. Am J Gastroenterol 1984;79:376–378.
41. Rhodes JM, Cockel R, Allan RN, et al: Colonic Crohn's disease and use of oral contraception. Br Med J 1984;288:595–596.

42. Korelitz BI: IBD in families, pregnancy, and childhood. Mt Sinai J Med (NY) 1983;50:181–186.
43. Vender RJ, Spiro HM: Inflammatory bowel disease and pregnancy. J Clin Gastroenterol 1982;4:231–249.
44. Mann J: Sickle cell haemoglobinopathies in England. Arch Dis Child 1981;56:676–683.
45. Alleyne R, Rauseo R, Serjeant G: Sexual development and fertility of Jamaican female patients with homozygous sickle cell disease. Arch Intern Med 1981;141:1295–1297.
46. Phebus CK, Gloninger MF, Maciak BJ: Growth patterns by age and sex in children with sickle cell disease. J Pediatr 1984;105:28–33.
47. Platt OS, Rosenstock W, Espeland MA: Influence of sickle hemoglobinopathies on growth and development. N Engl J Med 1984;311:7–12.
48. Westney LS, Callender CO, Stevens J, et al: Successful pregnancy with sickle cell disease and renal transplantation. Obstet Gynecol 1984;63:752–755.
49. Siris ES, Leventhal BG, Vaitukaites JL: Effects of childhood leukemia and chemotherapy on puberty and reproductive function in girls. N Engl J Med 1976;294:1143–1146.
50. Stillman RJ, Schinfield JS, Schiff I, et al: Ovarian failure in longterm survivors of childhood malignancy. Am J Obstet Gynecol 1981;139:62–66.

Index